Praise for Getting Ahead of ADHD

"As a parent who has read every book on the subject, I tried everything to help my son with ADHD. I made him feel like a lab rat and wasted time, energy, and money. If I could turn back time, this one book would sit on my nightstand. It is so nice to have a vision for a bright future alongside realistic, meaningful actions we can take right now. *Getting Ahead of ADHD* gives me the confidence and tools I need to make wise decisions."
—*Marie B., Oregon*

"How can you stay abreast of the rapidly growing research base on ADHD and its treatment, when even clinical professionals can't keep up? Simple— read this book! Dr. Nigg is a foremost clinical scientist with a talent for making complex ideas digestible. He explains what is currently known about the causes of ADHD, and, more important, offers numerous insights and recommendations for how to find the best treatment for your unique child."
—*Russell A. Barkley, PhD, ABPP, ABCN, author of*
Taking Charge of ADHD, Third Edition

"Thank you, Dr. Nigg! As a parent of a child with ADHD, I found this book tremendously valuable as well as enjoyable to read. It condenses the best current research into practical advice. For example, we've restricted the amount of added sugar in our family's diet and see a noticeable reduction in my child's irritability. I will definitely recommend this book to other parents who are looking for expert guidance."
—*Laura S., Michigan*

"Dr. Nigg presents a new understanding of ADHD that reveals how both genes and environment shape the disorder. He reviews the pros and cons of diet, exercise, and other novel treatments, helping you choose among a wide range of options for your child. Misinformation about ADHD abounds—this book separates facts from fiction."
—*Stephen V. Faraone, PhD, Distinguished Professor of Psychiatry*
and of Neuroscience and Physiology, State University
of New York Upstate Medical University

"This refreshingly commonsense book is outstanding in several ways—it is timely, relevant, comprehensive, balanced, and practical."
—*L. Eugene Arnold, MD, MEd, Department of Psychiatry*
and Behavioral Health (Emeritus), The Ohio State University
College of Medicine

GETTING AHEAD OF ADHD

Getting Ahead of ADHD

What Next-Generation Science Says about Treatments That Work—and How You Can Make Them Work for Your Child

Joel T. Nigg, PhD

THE GUILFORD PRESS
New York   London

Copyright © 2017 The Guilford Press
A Division of Guilford Publications, Inc.
370 Seventh Avenue, Suite 1200, New York, NY 10001
www.guilford.com

Printed in the United States of America

This book is printed on acid-free paper.

Last digit is print number: 9   8   7   6   5   4   3   2   1

Library of Congress Cataloging-in-Publication Data is available from the publisher.

ISBN 978-1-4625-2493-8 (paperback) — ISBN 978-1-4625-3032-8 (hardcover)

Contents

Acknowledgments

This book is the product of my perception that the latest emerging scientific ideas about ADHD reach parents and families too slowly. I hope those who have asked me for this type of information will find it useful.

No book is possible without the help of many different people in direct and indirect ways. Too numerous to name are the colleagues, students, and families who over the years have helped me refine my thinking and decide on the value of writing a trade book on this topic. I have tried to credit within the book many of the scientists and clinicians whose work has increased my understanding, although I am sure I have overlooked some who deserved mention.

However, a few individuals deserve specific thanks for their help with this book: Kitty Moore of The Guilford Press was inexhaustibly patient with multiple ideas and false starts before everything clicked. Christine Benton was superlative as line editor, advisor, reality check—and offered a perfect balance of candor and pragmatic encouragement. Both were exemplary in their professionalism, solution-oriented approach to snags, and good cheer. Keith Cheng, MD, and Kyle Johnson, MD, offered invaluable critique and comment on treatments and sleep, respectively. Katherine Holton, PhD, and Jeanette Johnstone, PhD, assisted in prior writings on which sections of the nutrition chapter rely.

To everyone, and to those not named who have encouraged and taught me, thank you, and good health.

GETTING AHEAD OF ADHD

Introduction

ADHD is the most widely studied disorder affecting children. Why then do parents still have so many questions about it? If you have a child with this condition or a related one, you've already benefited from how research evidence amassed over several decades has informed diagnosis and treatment. But everywhere you turn you still run into conflicting reports, controversies, debates, and claims about the latest "breakthrough" treatments or revelations about the "real" cause of this prevalent and challenging disorder. This is especially true for alternative interventions like diet or exercise; reliable information on these popular alternatives is much harder to come by relative to information on standard care via medicine or counseling.

A big reason for this confusing array of information and misinformation is that our scientific understanding of ADHD is rapidly changing. A more complex picture is emerging that offers you an opportunity to make a big difference in your child's health and happiness—and that of your whole family—both now and into the future. This is obviously great news, as long as you can sort fact from fiction. There's a lot to sift through, and it evolves every day.

The goal of this book is to present a clear explanation of what "next-generation" science tells us about ADHD—particularly a new understanding of how it is caused and the role of environmental influences. In the following pages I hope to put to rest some persistent myths and tell you what reliable research reveals and what we're still studying. I'll help you look at the controversies and claims with a discerning eye and form a solid idea of what kind of help is most likely to actually help your child.

1

What you'll read in this book is all founded on four major discoveries of recent years that are reshaping how we look at ADHD and are translating into practical new ways to help your child:

1. We now know that *there's a lot more to ADHD than inattention and/or hyperactivity*: The broader capacity of *self-regulation* is much more at the core of ADHD than these individual symptoms. Knowing something about what's involved in self-regulation opens up new ideas about how to understand your child's journey. It can help you finally comprehend why your child with ADHD doesn't act at all like the kid with ADHD next door or the one at the next desk over in the classroom.

2. *It's not all about genes*: Through growing interest in the interplay of genes and experiences and a new understanding of a phenomenon called *epigenetics,* we now know that genes are not destiny; how a genetic predisposition to ADHD (or anything else) is manifested in a child's functioning can be changed by the environment—that is, by the child's early and subsequent experiences. So in some ways the truly big news about ADHD today is that we've revived our interest in the role of the environment. This fascinating area of study tells us that factors like diet and screen use can have an impact after all (although no, they don't simply "cause" ADHD). Inheritance is not the only factor at the root of ADHD, and medication is not the only route to improvement for your child. The fact that genes are involved doesn't mean we can ignore the effects of all the input from the child's day-to-day world.

3. We know more than ever about *brain development and ADHD*: Until recently we thought that ADHD involved a handful of key brain areas; now we are beginning to see that ADHD involves how the brain is connecting and wiring itself across many regions. In fact, the way the entire brain organizes its communication patterns may be the key to understanding neurodevelopment and its disturbances or variations related to conditions like ADHD. We have a lot to learn in this complex area of study, but it's becoming clear that there are many potential routes to protecting children from ADHD and minimizing the symptoms.

4. We're learning more and more that *specific experiences have a powerful influence on the development of self-regulation, and therefore prob-*

ably on ADHD: Through epigenetic changes—including the power of sleep and exercise to grow the brain's network connections—these experiences affect both ADHD and other mental health conditions too.

These advances open up a world of ways that we can minimize the impact of a genetic predisposition to ADHD, not just in individual children but perhaps in generations to come as well.

In this book you'll learn about the latest science on how major factors in the environmental—stress, nutrition, exercise, sleep, and chemical pollution—affect ADHD, along with practical suggestions for using this information to minimize risk and boost protective factors. I'll walk you through the lifestyle choices that may be best for your child and help you understand which standard treatments and which alternatives make the most sense from the perspective of the new science. In the end, I hope you'll emerge from this book empowered with new understanding, new strategies, and new hope for your child's future.

How to Use This Book

In Chapters 1 and 2 you'll get the new science—how we now understand self-regulation of attention, emotion, and behavior, what we mean by epigenetics, and how it's involved in brain development. This is the foundation of the rest of the book, so I suggest that everyone read these two chapters. After that, you'll find five chapters on individual lifestyle and experiential factors that affect ADHD, for good and for ill. These chapters offer the details on how changes in the environment can change how your child's brain grows and how inattention, executive functioning, and self-regulation develop. Take a look at the table of contents and read Chapters 3–7 in whatever order interests you. Each chapter explains the state-of-the-art science on topics from diet to sleep to screen media and pollutants and then translates the data into practical strategies you can consider applying to your family's household routines and your child's daily life to improve ADHD and make everyone happier and healthier. For most children struggling with self-regulation problems like ADHD, some type of professional help will be an important element in treatment, so in Chapter 8 you'll find the latest science on what works and what doesn't and how to identify reliable treatments and qualified professionals. In Chapter 9 I'll help you bring all of this new understanding together so that you can decide on a course of action that will offer your child the best outcome, and one that's not so hard on your family that the "cure" ends up worse than the "disease."

Meanwhile, here are some of the main areas of discussion informed enormously by next-generation science:

ADHD Is Not Quite What We Thought It Was

It's increasingly clear that ADHD is the extreme on a spectrum, in the same way that hypertension (high blood pressure) is the extreme on the continuum of blood pressure. And it's not just about attention, but about the broader capacity we call *self-regulation*. Self-regulation means the ability to adjust attention, emotion, thinking, and behavior to suit a particular situation and one's own goals and intentions. This ability, obviously barely present in infants, grows throughout childhood. It becomes complex during the adolescent passage and matures all the way into the twenties. In ADHD, self-regulation develops more slowly, matures later, and often fails to reach full capacity even in adulthood. As a result, individuals with ADHD struggle not just with attention and organization, and with being impulsive, but often as well with difficulty controlling their emotions, whether that involves anxiety or anger. Yet their own learning history means that different aspects of self-regulation stand out for different kids, because self-regulation involves thinking, behavior, and emotions. When we look at ADHD along this spectrum, it becomes pretty clear how a group of even twenty children with the diagnosis can seem more different than alike.

The spectrum idea clarifies how some children can seem to manage the typical symptoms of ADHD fairly well (at least when they have lots of support from parents and teachers) while others suffer serious impairments. Recent research helps explain why some people struggle terribly with ADHD, and why we should not ignore it or try to wait it out, by showing that *well-developed self-regulation is more important than IQ, parenting skills, or school in predicting life success*. It is related to everything from how much money people will earn, to how healthy they will be, to how long they will live. When self-regulation fails in an extreme way, as in some kids with ADHD, the results can be disastrous: school failure, drug addiction, divorce, employment failure, illness, injuries, and earlier death. Even when ADHD is not quite this severe, it is typically associated with ongoing struggles in terms of emotional control, conflict with other people, and difficulty and frustration in school and work settings. We now know that it is also associated with a range of poorer health outcomes. In fact, because ADHD is related to so many subsequent problems, its total public health impact is probably still underappreciated despite all the publicity it continues to attract.

This is why you are right to want to help your child with ADHD get better at managing her own emotions, thinking, and behavior. It's why learning as much as we can about the problem through reliable and current scientific research is so essential.

There Are More Ways to Help Your Child Than You Might Have Thought

The good news is that there's a lot you can do to change the odds. I'll try to help you sort through the valid choices throughout this book. This is not a one-size-fits-all problem by any means. Please keep in mind, however, that the ideas you'll find here are not meant to replace standard professional care but to supplement it and perhaps reduce your child's need for it. The value in standard professional care is itself sometimes overlooked. While we have a new appreciation of the limits of medication and other traditional treatments for ADHD, they remain crucial for many children, and in this book I offer a few tips for how to get the most out of mainstream treatment to supplement what you'll find covered more comprehensively in other books (listed in the Resources at the end of this book). Here my focus is mainly on lifestyle and environment, which are addressed insufficiently in most books on ADHD.

From that angle, we'll be looking at a raft of common questions: Which self-help strategies work? Are any of the new "breakthroughs" real or are they "snake oil"? Will diet help? Is toxic pollution causing ADHD?

Are alternative treatments worth exploring? ADHD is "big business." It's easy to spend money on false promises. This book should give you confidence in deciding where to put your limited time and money to maximize the payoff for your child, from low-tech alternatives like fish oil supplements to high-tech options like neurofeedback.

ADHD remains a contentious topic in part due the rapidly rising rates of diagnosis and prescription of stimulant medication for young children. Over 11 percent of children in the United States have now been identified as having ADHD by a health care professional, and some 7 percent are being treated with simulant medication—with much higher rates among boys in late childhood. These rates have risen dramatically just between 2006 and 2012. All this despite the best epidemiological evidence that the true prevalence of carefully diagnosed ADHD is around 3–4 percent with no true increase in prevalence in the past decade (although it's quite possible it was increasing in the decades before that).

You've undoubtedly heard claims that ADHD is "always" overdiagnosed or misdiagnosed. You may even have heard that as a disorder it doesn't actually exist. While many factors in society are driving the current state of affairs and the confusion surrounding it, insufficient scientific information about what ADHD really is remains at the root of inaccurate diagnosis and inadequate intervention strategies. With the scientific data emerging today, we can refine diagnosis and supplement medication treatment and behavior management techniques with additional tools that can help a lot of children.

What Causes ADHD Is More Complicated Than We Believed

Perhaps the most urgent question about ADHD is what causes it. The still-popular view that the problem is poor parenting was long ago discredited by science. Unfortunately, the important idea that subtle early brain injury could be involved was then dismissed prematurely. Instead, a genetic story took over and still prevails in the minds of most clinicians and researchers. That was based sensibly enough on dramatic discoveries from twin studies showing real genetic influences. But here, too, the science has moved on. It is now clear that while genetics are clearly crucial, the traditional genetic model is simplistic enough to mislead us. Chapter 2 briefly explains the new perspective of epigenetics, which is closely related to a concept called "gene × environment interaction." Epigenetics as I use it in this book means that experiences can create stable, enduring—yet potentially reversible—changes in gene expression. These enduring changes in biology help us understand in a new way the importance of early life and ongoing stress, diet, exercise, and other influences. Not only can a child's environment, starting in the womb, steer development toward ADHD, but new, corrective, or healing experiences can restore healthier levels of gene expression. Much of this book is devoted to helping you see just where we are on this interesting, and largely underrecognized, frontier of science as it relates to ADHD.

One of the important strengths of science is that it evolves; it self-corrects; new knowledge supplants old knowledge. Seventy-five years ago, most experts did not think genetics was a major contributor to mental illness. A "naive environmentalism" ruled. Between 1960 and 2000 it became clear that we needed to take into account a major role for genes in ADHD and other mental disorders. But the pendulum swung too far—for many reasons. A genetic story was appealing; it felt safely grounded in rock-solid biology and had been successful in explaining other diseases in the past. (For example, insights from genetics revolutionized our understanding of the causes and treatments for intellectual disability in the second half of the twentieth century.) And it was easy, though logically incorrect, to think that because medication seemed to control ADHD symptoms, the disorder is biologically determined.

But science kept going. We realized through studies over the life span of individuals that medications didn't cure ADHD; they only controlled the symptoms (at least partially). And even that effect often seemed to "wear off" after a few years. Coincidentally, we also learned that we weren't in fact "solving" ADHD with genetics alone. The expected breakthroughs didn't occur. We began to realize that genes aren't the entire story, and that enduring yet potentially modifiable changes in how genes work are caused by early-life experiences—such as stress or diet—that change brain and behavior. Development is always the joint interplay of genetics and environment. This is the revolution that helped inspire the ideas in this book.*

What Do I Mean by "Science"?

Throughout the book, we will pay special attention to the highest-quality scientific evidence. I'll help you understand the different types of research studies so you know why I consider some data more reliable than others and so you can make your own judgments about future research reports. Here are the terms you'll encounter:

Meta-analysis. This means that all the studies on a question are combined in one "super analysis" to answer a question about how effective something is. A major development in the last few years is that today the methods of these analyses are widely known and used. For the first time we have summary data on almost all our questions rather than relying on isolated studies alone. The reliability of findings from meta-analysis depends on the size, quality, and number of individual studies being pooled, but it is still generally much better than insights from one study.

Systematic Reviews. These are similar to meta-analyses but often rely on an evaluation of highest-quality versus lowest-quality studies.

Randomized Controlled Trials. In these powerful experiments, an intervention—such as exercise or diet—is assigned at random to one group of children while another group of children is assigned at random to a different intervention. In the best design, neither the child nor the experimenter knows which child got which treatment (that is the meaning of a "double blind" study). For example, half the children might drink a milk shake in a black container with food coloring in it, while the

---

*One scientific dispute is whether the epigenetic approach is in fact revolutionary. It's not revolutionary in one sense—epigenetic effects have been known about for decades. But what is revolutionary is the recognition that a great deal of human disease, particularly complex problems like psychiatric and behavioral disorders, probably involves epigenetic mechanisms. The epigenetics of human brain and behavior is still a new and in many ways revolutionary approach to the field.

other half get a milk shake that tastes the same but has no food coloring. In a random assignment, there is no way to explain effects other than that they are caused by the one variable that was controlled—such as food coloring in this example. Randomization removes all other possible causes. The power and magic of experimental random assignment is that these studies can show that one thing caused another, not just that the two happened to appear together.

Prospective Studies. This means the outcome follows the treatment or the exposure in time. For example, children might be recruited at birth, and their early-life exposure to stress or toxic chemicals measured, and then some years later their behavior is studied and they are assessed for ADHD. While it doesn't prove cause, this type of study still is more powerful than simply looking at both toxic chemical exposure and ADHD symptoms at a single point in time, when we don't know what came first.

Whole-Population Studies. Many studies of ADHD have used what are called convenience samples—such as children coming to a clinic or volunteers from a local community. It is often difficult to generalize from these locales to other locales—although meta-analyses can help. In recent years, powerful computers have enabled the United States and several other countries to obtain representative samples of the entire population of a region or nation using large databases. These tell us how "real" effects are in size and importance compared to smaller studies. Small studies can overestimate the true size of an effect, while large population studies can help make that estimate more accurate. However, large population studies often have to settle for somewhat limited measurement of ADHD and other variables, leading to questions about how valid they are. To get a complete picture, we would ideally look not only at whole-population studies, but also at meta-analyses, randomized trials, and in-depth studies of local populations. I've tried to draw from the best of these approaches.

I'll get into more detail about the "gold standard" for reliable research studies as we go along, but it's also important to know that how much evidence clinicians and scientists require to find an effect valid depends on what the intervention is. If we're looking at something that is generally safe and healthy overall, such as moderate exercise, we require less evidence to recommend it. On the other hand, we will scrutinize much more carefully ideas that are expensive or risky, such as some of the new high-tech treatments.

Where We—and the Science—Are Headed

The fields of psychiatry, clinical and developmental psychology, medicine, and neuroscience are dynamic and rapidly changing. We now are seeing that, just as ADHD is not a myth, not caused by parents or teachers, but also not simply genetic, the brain keeps redesigning itself and adapting with time, and the body and mind are intimately connected. My aim here is to help you see this trend and take advantage of it. To quote the great hockey player Wayne Gretzky, I want to help readers "skate to where the puck is going," to take advantage of expert knowledge not only in its most cutting-edge form at the moment but also as I perceive it soon will become. I will try to help you gauge what future science may show us, extrapolating from trends in the most recent science.

You should take away from this book a fresh and hopeful understanding of how ADHD develops and how it can change. The new paradigm will, I hope, free you from self-blame but also empower you and better equip you to balance the "best of the old" and the "best of the new" in ADHD science for your child.

1

A New Understanding
of ADHD

You probably know that ADHD means *attention-deficit/hyperactivity disorder*. And you might have found out online that children with this condition have serious problems paying attention, sitting still, taking their turn, or finishing what they start. This pattern typically starts early in life and remains stable, although some individuals seem to have a slightly later onset and others seem to "recover" in adolescence and adulthood. If your child has been diagnosed with ADHD, the effects are familiar to you. But what is ADHD? Why do so many of the features of children with ADHD not seem like deficits in attention? Why are some kids labeled with ADHD even though they aren't hyperactive? You might be asking yourself, "Why was my child diagnosed with ADHD when his main problem is anger?" Before we delve into the new thinking about what causes ADHD and how this can give you hope for change, it's important to understand how the different manifestations of ADHD are connected.

Where experts once saw ADHD as a problem of attention, and then of executive functioning, the picture has evolved again in recent years, and now we can best understand it as a problem with *self-regulation*. This shift gives us a perspective that is both more complex and more powerful. Self-regulation involves a half dozen processes or capabilities that, when any one of them doesn't develop properly, can create the appearance of ADHD. Similar to executive functioning but broader, the capacity of self-regulation helps us understand the breadth of challenges faced by

children (and adults) with ADHD as well as the very important variations that occur in the disorder. It also helps us recognize that many of
the frustrating behaviors associated with ADHD are just as frustrating
to the individuals with ADHD themselves, seeming to occur before they
can get a handle on what is going on. However, in children and adults,
this frustration can get turned outward, toward blaming others for their
own problems. Together, these new perspectives can clear the way for
new hope and new solutions to help children with ADHD.

What Is Self-Regulation?

Self-regulation means the capacity to optimize our behavior, thinking
and attention, and emotional experience and expression. Note that we
say *optimize*—self-regulation doesn't just mean the ability to suppress or
inhibit an impulse or control an emotional outburst, although that's part
of it. It also means the ability to *activate*—or energize and persist—when
needed.

So one of the first misconceptions about ADHD is that it's only a
deficiency in the ability to inhibit (or that it's really just impulsivity).
Now, not being able to inhibit is indeed a core feature of ADHD. Kids
with ADHD blurt out what they shouldn't say, have a hard time resisting
temptation, and act in ways that they regret. But they also have trouble
activating—getting started, initiating, and maintaining effort over time.
Both inhibiting and activating are part of regulating. Finally, they have
trouble fine-tuning. For example, even in studies in which children are
asked to press with steady force on a plate, they have trouble holding
consistent pressure—it varies from too high to too low. They go too
slowly when they have to go fast, and too fast when they have to go
slowly. All of this together is self-regulation. If you think of ADHD as a
self-regulating problem, rather than an
attention or inhibition problem, it is a bit
easier to see the connection between seemingly opposite behaviors.

> One reason for ADHD's variability is that it's not just a problem with inhibition; it's also a problem with activation.

Take ten-year-old Jenny as an example.
Her mother reported, with some puzzle-

ment, that "I can see why she has ADHD because she can't focus on her homework for more than two minutes without me standing right there to make her do it. But then she gets so focused on her doll collection that I can't get her to break away from it to do something else. And she can lock on to a video game for hours! So it seems like she can pay attention when she wants to." The explanation for this apparent contradiction is that Jenny cannot *optimize* her attention. She can't really control it. Instead, her attention controls her. She can't focus on her homework when she needs to. Her attention is captured by her doll collection or the video game, and she can't break away without a struggle. In a way, Jenny isn't entirely free, because she can't put her attention where her ultimate goals would suggest. (Caution—if the only time attention is a problem is when a child is doing schoolwork, it's important to rule out a learning disability.)

All of self-regulation is connected. Kids who can't focus their attention also frequently cannot get a handle on behavior. This is why classic ADHD looks like inattention plus impulsivity (and in young children hyperactivity, or in older individuals extreme restlessness). It's also why problems getting a handle on emotions commonly plague kids with ADHD as well. Yet the degree of these different problems varies like a rainbow among kids with ADHD, with different profiles common.

> *Self-regulation applies to a child's thoughts, actions, and emotions, which is why the typical picture of ADHD includes problems with mental focus (inattention) and problems controlling behavior (impulsivity).*

What Is Impulsivity?

Impulsivity is one consequence of weak self-regulation—in the arena of *action*. Impulsivity means habitually and nonreflectively responding to the immediate trigger or the immediate payoff, regardless of whether it's ultimately the best choice. The hallmark of dysfunctional impulsivity is inability to adjust how impulsive we are to fit the circumstances. For example, an average adult without ADHD may be quite impulsive and spontaneous at a party with friends, but then be planful and controlled at work or when dealing with more serious matters. A typically developing child without development problems like ADHD may be spontaneous and excitable on a vacation but able to settle in to calm, focused work at school or relaxed calm behavior at dinner. ADHD is characterized by inability to get out of the spontaneous, excitable, or "highly reactive" state, even when the situation calls for it.

Because of this problem with self-regulation of action, seven-year-old Dan was in constant trouble at school. When the child next to him stacked some blocks on the table, Dan knocked them down for the thrill of it, before he even thought. Likewise, eighteen-year-old Maria was unhappy with herself. Friday evening she had baked a cake for a friend's birthday party the next day. She was proud of herself for managing to bake the cake. It looked good, so she decided to have a little piece. In fact, it was *really* good, and before she knew it she had eaten a third of the cake. Now she was really unhappy because she had eaten too much and the cake was not fit to take to the party as a gift. People with ADHD often make others mad, disappoint themselves, and are at risk for addiction, because when they have an idea, feel a desire, or sense a craving, it pours into action almost by itself. They have trouble interrupting the path from internal thought or feeling to action. This is poor action control or poor impulse control.

Here's a lighthearted example. In a movie called *The Shaggy Dog*, the comedian Tim Allen plays a man who sometimes turns into a dog involuntarily. He retains his human awareness—but now has a dog's instincts. As a result, he is ruefully impulsive. He narrates his thoughts during the dog scenes. One incident in the movie perfectly illustrates impulsivity and disinhibition. The humanly aware dog is in his house, where his teenage daughter thinks he is just the family dog. She and her boyfriend are in her bedroom preparing to "make out" on the bed. Disapproving of this, but being a dog, Allen tries to intervene by hanging out in the room and annoying the teenagers. The boyfriend picks up a toy bone to distract the dog. We hear a voice-over by Allen: "That's not going to work. I'm not going to fall for that! No way! I'm staying right here!" The kid then tosses the toy bone out into the hallway, where the shaggy dog immediately bolts for it, and then of course is quickly locked out of the bedroom by the two would-be lovers. In the next voice-over Allen, in a tone of exasperation, says, "I have to quit doing that!"

This is impulsivity—doing something for an immediate reward or trigger that defeats one's established goals. Doing, in a sense, the opposite of what one really wants to do. As in this example, dogs are impulsive when seen through human eyes: they react to the immediate moment without regard to any semblance of a long-term goal. In a much more serious vein, we see something similar in addiction. The alcoholic wants to be sober—but he also wants a drink. His immediate impulse and ultimate goal are in conflict. If he takes the drink, he satisfies his immediate craving but defeats his ultimate goal. Similarly, an individual with ADHD as a teen or adult may blurt out an inappropriate insult or flirtatious remark—even after resolving not to do this—and then immediately regret it. A typically developing individual without ADHD may have the same passing thought but suppress it and move on without acting on it.

Impulsivity—poor self-regulation of action—often results in a general style that is spontaneous and excitable. When spontaneous and excitable is the best approach, a child or adult with ADHD may do well. This is why some children with ADHD can be a lot of fun at a party or during a break from school. It's why some individuals with ADHD find a niche in the adult world where their style can succeed. I have seen adults, sometimes parents of children with ADHD, who have become salesmen, entertainers, or even entrepreneurs (assisted by organized teammates), working in settings where their active, high-energy, spontaneous style seems to fit and to complement others around them. But because they had ADHD, they could not adapt well to other settings—they struggled or failed in school, failed at jobs that required careful, quiet work, and had interpersonal problems and conflicts from not being able to adjust their tempo and style and not being able to stay organized or manage time. With ADHD, this spontaneous, immediate response style is practically always "on." Whether or not it is the right style for the situation becomes irrelevant. That's just a matter of luck (for a child) or of fortune and insight for an adult.

Impulsivity may work well where a high-energy, spontaneous, or self-directed style is a plus (such as in jobs in sales or entertainment, or requiring lots of physical energy), but because it's practically always switched on, it can cause trouble in other settings.

I should add that for some individuals the impulsive aspect of ADHD is severe enough that they never seem to be able to find the right niche. Our modern world doesn't provide enough of the right kind of niche, or their loss of self-regulation is too extreme for almost any niche without a lot of support. They need extra professional help, both as children and as adults.

What about ADD?

There is one important variation to explain right here—that is why many people ask what "ADD" means. Rhonda brought her eleven-year-old son Tyrone in for an evaluation. She had been told he had ADHD but said, "I just don't see it. Yes, he can't pay attention and he's very spaced out. He zones out whenever I talk to him, and his friends even tease him for being a 'space cadet.' The teacher is concerned that he's not following in class. But he's not hyperactive in the least! Just the opposite! He's laid back, even lazy. He'll sit around the house and not do anything. It doesn't make any sense to call him ADHD!"

Rhonda is right: ADHD is not a very helpful term for kids who are not hyperactive. But the picture here makes sense when we think of ADHD as a problem in self-regulation and remember that regulating means *optimizing*. Some kids with ADHD are not overactive. They are *under*active. They seem to be slower than normal, low in energy, even lethargic—yet very inattentive. Some people use the now-discarded term ADD for these children. This is not an official medical term; it is an older term for ADHD.

This profile has been called instead *sluggish cognitive tempo*, referring to children who are spaced out, experience frequent mind wandering, and easily get tired. They are prone to depression and anxiety, although not all of them develop those problems. While this is not yet an official diagnostic label, we're seeing more and more data supporting its existence, and we're likely to see increasing interest in it.

Such children have a different self-regulation problem: poor *activation*. They can't get activation up to where it belongs—cannot initiate or raise their level of activity. They are too low and slow, even when it is not useful. Like impulsive and overactive children, they have poor self-regulation of their action but on the opposite side. You might be able to relate to this by thinking of those times you wanted to go exercise but just couldn't get yourself out the door or wanted to get out of bed on a rainy morning but just couldn't summon the necessary willpower.

While experts continue to explore whether these sluggish children have a variant of ADHD or a distinct condition, for our purposes we can follow current practice and see these children as a different but related variation of the "self-regulation disorder" that, for historical reasons, is called ADHD.

So at this point you can see that poor self-regulation can mean that attention is overfocused or underfocused. Poor self-regulation of action means that action can be habitually impulsive and spontaneous, without the ability to *inhibit*. It can also be habitually underactive and slow, without the ability to *activate*. These both fall under the umbrella of inability to *optimize* to the situation.

> *Poor self-regulation affects both ends of the continuum—overfocused or underfocused attention, poor inhibition or poor activation.*

Why Is My Child So Anxious and So Angry? Is That Part of ADHD?

Perhaps the most important insight about self-regulation from recent science is that, because self-regulation is all connected, children with ADHD typically have problems regulating their *emotion*, too. This symptom still confuses many parents, and also confuses many clinicians because they have not connected it to a "global self-regulation disorder." I was asked to consult on the case of Mike, an eight-year-old boy with ADHD. Mike was inattentive and impulsive. But what bothered his parents, and made his doctor unsure of the diagnosis, was that Mike seemed so moody. He could be confident and outgoing. But as soon as he was told he had lost a privilege due to poor behavior, he might start to cry. When he had to sit still at a desk and work, he might work for a few minutes, then he would shout, "I can't stand this!" at the top of his lungs. When it was time to go to the doctor, he worried about it all day long. "What if he gives me a shot? What time are we going? Will it take very long?" He had trouble sleeping the night before and had a tantrum when it was time to get in the car. Assuming that sitting for the schoolwork was nothing unusual; assuming the doctor is not too mean; assuming Mike is not actually depressed (an important rule-out for children who are moody and have tantrums), all of this is part of poor self-regulation of emotion, and part of the ADHD syndrome—even though not part of the official diagnostic criteria.

Mike's emotions are all over the place, and he cannot get a handle on them. He overreacts emotionally to everything—at least that's how it seems to other people. In fact, he may be having emotions that are fairly typical—many children are disappointed when they lose a privilege, restless when they have to sit too long at a desk, or a little nervous when they go to the doctor. But Mike's emotions are more intense. It's as if there is no governor on the system. His emotions take over, and he seems unable to regulate them very well. This seeming emotionality may not be a separate emotional disorder. It may simply be part of the ADHD syndrome—a syndrome of poor self-regulation. ADHD includes self-regulation of attention, of action, and of emotions. This is very different from depression, which is a problem of regulation of mood (often outside the realm of self-control), and anxiety, a problem of self-regulation of anxious thoughts. In a primary mood disorder, we are facing a particular imbalance in regulation of positive affect (in the case of depression), or negative affect (worry or fear, in the case of anxiety). In the case of ADHD, we face a general breakdown in self-regulation of action as well as cognition and often, secondarily, of emotion.

When it comes to emotion, we again see significant variation. Recent research from my laboratory and those of my colleagues, published in 2014 and 2015, suggests that ADHD has subgroups in terms of emotional style, with different physiological responses and different brain imaging responses. Yet all the groups have similar degrees of ADHD symptoms. One group seems to have pretty typical emotional responses. These kids might be spacey, inattentive, and maybe not overactive. Their emotions are low key and they don't get super angry or super amped up. They are similar to the inattentive, underactive children we described above. However, there are exceptions—some of these emotionally typical children also have the full ADHD syndrome. Somehow, their emotional regulation came together even though they haven't yet been able to regulate their attention or action.

The second group has trouble mainly with regulating positive emotions. They are very excitable, very active, and very outgoing. But they aren't flexible in this style, and so they get into trouble by overdoing it and pushing too far. They may get angry when they can't get what they want or think they deserve. They seem to have a relatively mild form of ADHD in which things go okay over time, despite some trouble in school and at home, and they are able to manage with support, and some get better as they get older.

The final group has trouble mainly with regulating their negative emotions. They get very unhappy and also have anger outbursts and tantrums over minor annoyances. Once they "lose it" in a tantrum, they can't settle down. They stay upset for a long time. They aren't very socially confident, and although they are hyperactive, they aren't quite as overactive or energetic as the "positive emotion" group. These children seem to have a different pattern of brain activity than the others. They also are at risk for developing mood problems—many had a new anxiety disorder, mood disorder, or defiant disorder when we followed them up two years later. These emotional groups predicted how well children would do over time more accurately than the measures currently used by professionals. We need more evidence to change the way children are evaluated, but this research does help clarify both that emotion regulation is important in ADHD and that kids with ADHD differ in important ways in their cognitive and emotional profile. While these groups, like other ways of subdividing kids with ADHD, are not absolute, and a child's profile can change or, in some cases, seem to be a mix of these profiles, this idea works pretty well and provides a way to begin to think about natural variation in the ADHD experience.

> Children with ADHD can have trouble regulating either positive or negative emotions.

So self-regulation means self-regulation of attention and cognition (what I think about, what I focus on), of action (what I do and don't do), and of emotion (how I express my emotions and how I deal internally with strong emotions). In ADHD, the different kinds of self-regulation are variations on the same core syndrome, while in mood disorders there is primary dysregulation of one of the emotion systems.

Isn't "Poor Self-Regulation" Just a Fancy Term for "Lazy"?

This may be the biggest misconception that we can fall into. Here's where it's helpful to understand a few of the components of self-regulation. Self-regulation isn't carried out by a little engineer sitting in our brain. Instead, it's accomplished by teamwork from different functions in the brain. If any part of the team doesn't do its job, self-regulation can break down. Science in recent years has begun to be able to separate and measure these components or team members. Who are they?

The Brain's Self-Regulation Team

ALERTNESS/DETECTION

The first is called *detection*. It's also called alertness. This is the capacity to notice a signal from our environment. This is only partly under our control. For example, you can sit up and really watch to notice when something is about to happen. You can drive the car and stay very alert to watch for an unfamiliar turn. But you don't have total control of this capacity. When you are very tired or distracted, you may drive past that turn despite your best effort to watch for it. Your capacity to notice is weakened. For kids with ADHD, breakdown in detection/alertness can cause them to seem like they aren't listening or aren't paying attention. See the box on the facing page for experiments that use brain electrical recordings to prove this possibility—showing that children with ADHD miss relevant cues in their environment.

This system helps us see why stimulant medication can actually "calm" a child with ADHD.

To understand this, think of alertness not as how alert or aroused the *person* is, but how aroused or awake the *brain* is—some people use the phrase "sleepy brain" for ADHD to convey this idea. This is not a bad way to think of it. A sleepy brain can lead to a poorly focused, even overactive individual. The advanced part of the brain, called the cortex, handles most of what we experience as conscious thinking and awareness, as well as most of our planned motor behaviors. Its level of arousal or alertness is called *cortical arousal*. While you've heard that ADHD involves brain

HOW WE DETECT INCONSISTENT ATTENTION IN THE BRAIN

In ADHD the brain doesn't consistently fire correctly when a warning signal appears. One reason that kids with ADHD might misbehave is that they are failing to pick up relevant cues in their surroundings. A group of researchers in Germany has led the way on this discovery. In a series of experiments, children with and without ADHD completed a computer task in which they had to respond to a target, except when they got a warning signal not to. During the task, experimenters recorded millisecond-by-millisecond brain waves coming through the scalp, using very sensitive electrodes placed on the scalp. These electrodes detected a pattern across millions of neurons in the cortex firing in sync in response to the computer stimulus. Typically developing children showed a "spike" of brain activity about 200 milliseconds after the computer warning, indicating that the brain was detecting the signal and sending it forward for advanced processing. In kids with ADHD, this burst of activity in the brain was either missing or much smaller. This indicates that the warning was not registering in the brain even though they were looking at the screen. This weakness might be overcome by making the signal easier to notice, increasing the child's brain energy state (as discussed in Chapter 3 on food and Chapter 4 on exercise), or allowing more time to process the signal. Parenting and teaching suggestions on how to give instructions to children with ADHD increasingly draw on this insight.

WANT TO READ MORE ABOUT THIS STUDY?

McLoughlin, G., Albrecht, B., Banaschewski, T., Rothenberger, A., Brandeis, D., Asherson, P., et al. (2009). Performance monitoring is altered in adult ADHD: A familial event-related potential investigation. *Neuropsychologia, 47*(14), 3134–3142.

---

chemistry, it also involves brain electrical signaling. Cortical arousal can be measured with electrodes on the scalp that detect the electrical activity being continuously produced by the brain. Using these signals, and some sophisticated math, scientists sort the signals into "slow-wave" and "fast-wave" forms, just like we can use a prism to sort light into long and short wavelengths. When we are sleepy and not dreaming, we have lots of slow-wave (or long wavelength) activity. When our mind is alert, we have a balance of slow-wave and fast-wave (or "short-wave") activity. EEGs using scalp electrodes have shown that many children with ADHD have excessive slow-wave activity in their brain-wave patterns while awake. This implies that their brain is underaroused.

An important point about cortical arousal (and thus alertness) is that *more is not always better.* A panicked child is no more able to focus than a lethargic child. If your brain is at extremely low arousal, you are asleep, or in a coma. If it is at maximum arousal, you have a panic attack or a seizure. Similarly, if you are too "laid back," you'll miss important things that are happening. When you are too anxious (too aroused), you can't think straight either. Thus, part of the challenge in ADHD is that the brain does not effectively regulate arousal or alertness. As a result, one child is overaroused, another is underaroused, but both are poorly equipped for the situation they are dealing with.

In ADHD, a child's brain may be overaroused or underaroused— but in both cases the child is not well equipped for the situation at hand.

In recent years my colleagues and I, and other researchers, have also evaluated arousal in the laboratory using heart rate measures. With sophisticated analysis of the heartbeat using an electrocardiograph (ECG) and another type of measurement called impedance we can partially separate the signals from the sympathetic and the parasympathetic nervous systems. The sympathetic nervous system gives us an index of physiological arousal that is related, through various nerve connections from heart to brain, to brain arousal. We can clearly see that some kids with ADHD are overaroused: they are too excitable, or too angry, or too sensitive to be effective in a situation. Others are underaroused: they tend to be indifferent or apathetic toward situations around them and can seem antisocial or cold toward others as a result. (Caution: Some children truly are cold or indifferent toward others, an important problem requiring further evaluation.)

Thus Molly, who is a worrier, might struggle on a test because she is too overaroused (for example, too anxious or too excited) to focus. Katie, on the other hand, can flunk a test because she is too underaroused to move quickly through

The optimal state of arousal is "relaxed alert." Knowing whether your child's brain tends to be overaroused or underaroused can provide a key to helping her succeed.

the material and thus gets only half of it done. So we want our child's brain arousal not to be "high" or "low" but "just right" for the situation at hand. Psychologically, to function best, we don't want to be on "red alert," nor do we want to be "asleep at the switch." We want to be "relaxed alert."

INFORMATION FILTERING AND ACCUMULATION

The second "team member" in the brain's regulation system is called information filtering/accumulation. In an everyday sense, we filter when we try to concentrate and when we ignore distraction. For example, at a party, you might be able to listen to what your friend is saying even though three other conversations are happening around you. You can filter those out—if your friend is particularly charismatic, you may do so almost effortlessly; if your friend is dull, it may take all your mental effort. However, there is another kind of filtering that happens more automatically all the time: when we look at a situation, we have to automatically "read it" after we detect it. Let's say you're having a conversation with someone you don't know very well, and he makes a surprising comment. You can't tell if he is trying to be friendly or if there is a hint of hostility in the remark. Over the course of that split second, your brain samples the environment hundreds of times to detect change and to compare signals with your own mental maps of reality to see if the pattern coming into the brain is more likely to fit "friendly" or "hostile." Kids with ADHD actually seem to filter distraction well in simple computer experiments, but they seem to check and accumulate information inefficiently or slowly, leading them to judge what they are sensing slowly and inaccurately.

You may have heard about brain waves being used in diagnostic tests for ADHD and in "neurofeedback" treatments for it. We'll talk about the scientific evidence for and against those treatments in Chapters 5 and 8. For now, the important point about brain waves is that they tell us self-regulation very probably has something to do with the frequency of brain oscillations as we sample the environment and compare input with internal models or "predictions" of reality.

A partial analogy here is radar. A radar screen pings the air frequently and compares what bounces back with what bounced back last time. By comparing the two, it detects change and motion. In humans, the visual system oscillates about 60 hertz (60 times in one second or once every 16.6 milliseconds). It's on this principle that we perceive motion when a television screen displays sequential images at about 70 hertz—our system doesn't "refresh" fast enough to detect the series of still pictures. Other brain and body systems oscillate at other frequencies. The human brain has multiple oscillation patterns operating at the same time, among different collections of neurons. These electrical oscillations are, in part, probably the result of brain networks comparing inputs, in effect comparing patterns with recent perception as well as with mental maps or mental predictions of what should be "out there."

That is a process of information accumulation and filtering. Your brain has to pick up each piece of information, look at it, and put it in pile A or pile B. It has to happen quickly, because you can only stare at your ambiguous colleague so long before you have to decide how to respond. After enough "votes" come in, your brain has enough information to make its decision.

We often do this accumulation and filtering automatically and easily, such as when we look at a clear picture (driving our car on a familiar road on a clear day; laughing at an obvious joke from a good friend). We do it with difficulty when the scene is ambiguous (driving on an unfamiliar road on a rainy night; sorting how to interpret an ambiguous remark from a stranger). We might have noticed everything (detection: we saw what there was to see on the sign; we picked up every nuance in the stranger's voice and facial expression), but we struggle to discern what it was—did that sign say speed limit 50 or 55? Did that individual mean to be friendly or hostile? Was that Hollywood supermodel smiling at me, or the VIP standing next to me? (Just checking to see if you're with me.) If you have the luxury to stop and stare at the sign, after a moment the picture might resolve itself. You'll see that it's one or the other. Your brain will accumulate enough samples of the picture to get a majority vote of signals.

But sometimes the picture only partially resolves, or time runs out, and you have to guess. If your brain is efficient at filtering, sorting, and accumulating in its hundreds of millisecond samples of reality, you will make mostly accurate guesses. If you have a major psychotic illness, your brain makes many wrong guesses about the information sorting.

For kids with ADHD, that brain "perceptual voting" process is inefficient. This means that even if they detect information, they are slow to sort it in their brain, as noted above: when events happen fast (as in a social interaction), they more often guess wrong about what is going on when they have to act. As an analogy, when you drive by a road sign in heavy traffic and can't slow down to study it, you have to guess. You might guess wrong, but you can't keep studying the sign. You just have to guess. A lot of situations may be that way for kids with ADHD. Their brain is accumulating and sorting information from their environment more slowly than the situation requires, as if the brain is cycling more slowly to "sample" its world. Perhaps the brain needs ten samplings to reach a decision threshold on a given ambiguous picture. That takes the average child 160 milliseconds. But if the child with ADHD has less efficient or, in effect, "noisier" sampling, with the equivalent of static from unfiltered information coming in, then she may need, say, fifteen cycles to get clarity—call it 240 milliseconds total. During learning, reading, complex behavior, or social interactions, that extra 80 milliseconds can be the difference between an astute and a misguided response. Another possibility is that the child with ADHD can also do it in ten samplings, but each oscillation takes 20 milliseconds instead of 16.5—so again, the processing is too slow. Picture a professional card dealer sorting cards by suit. She does it very fast. Now you try it. You'll go slower—because you will take a split second longer to recognize the suit before you decide which pile to put the card in. We can measure reaction times in the laboratory, and we can demonstrate this slower processing and response time in children with ADHD at about 20–40 milliseconds on very rapid tasks.

> The slow processing speed seen in ADHD makes it difficult to rapidly filter incoming information and make good decisions about the appropriate response in many day-to-day life situations.

Even while the child with ADHD is running at a slower "refresh rate" to evaluate a signal, the world doesn't slow down for her to study it. Her brain has to decide whether a child's joke was mean or playful, whether the teacher said the test was Tuesday or Thursday, whether the letter on the page is a *b* or a *d*. She has to guess before she has enough information, and therefore she more often guesses wrong. The science box on page 27 gives an example of how researchers know this can happen using mathematical models of decision making on computer tasks.

DELIBERATE CONTROL: OUTCOME

Only after detection and filtering/accumulation do we take action. (This all happens rapidly—within less than a second in normal behavior.) And it's really only at this last step that what we call "deliberate" action comes in. Here's where we "decide" consciously to inhibit, to check the swing as the ball breaks wide of the plate, to bite our tongue as we see the stranger smile and realize it was a friendly comment, or to say "bad" instead of "dad" while reading aloud. Only at that point do we activate—move, speak, or look. Here's where executive functioning comes into play— such as using working memory to solve difficult problems. These executive functions include:

1. Working memory—holding two or more things in mind at once while mentally manipulating one or more of them.
2. Inhibition—resisting doing something you are pulled to do for the sake of a later goal.
3. Interference control—resisting distracting thoughts.
4. Set shifting—seeing things from more than one point of view or approaching a problem a different way.

They are often called "top-down" operations because they depend on connections from the prefrontal cortex to other parts of the brain. If we have a goal or a focus in mind, based on top-down executive functions, that can shape or bias those "bottom-up" or automatic detection and filtering processes that we just mentioned. You may have noticed this, for example, if you were trying to decide what car to buy—suddenly you notice the qualities of other cars, things you ordinarily would not notice. Even so, we can't fully control what automatic filtering does or how well these automatic abilities work. That's one reason kids with ADHD sometimes just can't focus despite trying. Here, again, in the past decade several teams of scientists have helped to show that children with

THE IMPORTANCE OF EFFICIENT INFORMATION UPTAKE OR ACCUMULATION IN ADHD

A perennial challenge scientifically is to figure out how the brain actually makes decisions. The leading theories use computational models. They suggest that our brain uses an "information accumulator" that fires a signal when it reaches a threshold. The brain refreshes its visual perceptual signal about sixty times per second, while it has some cells oscillating much faster and some much slower to compare that signal to mental models of what it "thinks" is happening. Scientists know this from using single-cell recordings of different neurons in animals while they study a computer picture and decide what to do. In humans, these oscillations can be detected by various kinds of brain imaging. That model fits with what is known about how neural signals accumulate to fire the next neuron during information processing. The efficiency of information gain can now be mathematically modeled during simple computer experiments, and this has recently begun to be applied to children with ADHD by Cynthia Huang-Pollock and colleagues at Penn State and Sarah Karalunas and colleagues at Oregon Health & Science University. In a series of studies between 2012 and 2016, children with ADHD completed simple decision tasks. For example, they would watch a computer screen, and when a letter appeared they would press a key to indicate if it was an X or an O. The computer records the speed and accuracy of decision responses with millisecond accuracy over hundreds of trials. Researchers then conduct a detailed mapping of second-by-second, trial-by-trial responses using sophisticated mathematical models. The mathematical formulas are able to break down the errors and response times into distinct psychological components. These include "bias" (how much of a tendency you have to want to press the key or not press the key), "threshold" (how much information you require before deciding what the letter was), and "gain," or how efficient you are at accumulating information millisecond by millisecond against the "noise" of other activity in the mind and brain. Children with ADHD appear to have normal bias and normal threshold. Their reason for poor performance on the task appears to be inefficient information gain. This might be related to reduced speed of neural transmission (due to poorly developed myelin cells on neural axons), weak neural connections, or any number of environmental factors that might be addressed by methods detailed later in the book.

ADHD are not all alike in their cognitive profiles. At least as measured in the lab, problems with executive functions characterize some children, but other types of processing problems seem to characterize others.

Sometimes this top-down or controlled mode is limited in its capacity too. Why is this? One basic reason is that the controlled mode takes energy. Attention and willpower act like a muscle in some ways. It has a limited capacity, and then it tires out and needs time to recharge. As a result, we get tired when we have to focus attention on something difficult for very long or overcome a temptation using willpower. In the laboratory, people asked to focus on a boring display to find an occasional target letter get slower and less accurate as the minutes go by. Those who have to do mental math are less able to resist a piece of candy a few minutes later. The science box on the facing page gives more details on these interesting and still controversial studies.

Kids with ADHD seem to have less of this mental resource or capacity. Because controlled attention takes effort, it wears out. It wears out *faster* for kids with ADHD. So while Molly may be able to ignore her brother for fifteen minutes before she can't continue, Katie may make it for only one minute before the effort at concentration has exhausted her capacity.

This doesn't mean that all mental activity takes effort. No, just the opposite. In fact, the brain is always busy, doing background tuning and checking, even when we are just resting or daydreaming, and in an obvious way when we are sleeping and dreaming too. Clearly, at times the brain can run on "autopilot."

But it works in a different way when we have to focus our attention against competing distractions. Then we need to invest a certain kind of energy. This energy or capacity is finite—we can only process so much conscious information at one time, and after concentrating hard for too long, we start to feel tired of it. For this reason, the human mind has evolved to minimize the need for deliberate control or deliberate attention by allowing learned tasks and behaviors to be handed off to this autopilot. Because deliberate attention is not free, the brain has learned to conserve it. Whenever possible, the "controller" shuts down and work is delegated to automatic subroutines of thinking, responding, and acting. We see this when we drive home from work, mind wandering. We

WHY DO SCIENTISTS THINK THAT TOP-DOWN CONTROL TIRES OUT?

A series of experiments by Roy Baumeister and his colleagues at Florida State University in recent years have yielded fascinating results. In classic experiments several years ago, participants completed two tasks. The first task demanded a lot of self-control in one sphere (emotion, or attention, or action). The second demanded self-control too, but in a different sphere (emotion, attention, or action). In one example, the first task was to watch an emotional film without showing any emotion. The control group was allowed to show emotion. After that, everyone in both groups had to squeeze a grip lever as long as possible. Those who had to control their emotions on the film task gave up sooner on the grip task. In a more recent study, the researchers randomly assigned college students to write a difficult essay (avoid words with *a* or *n* in them) or an easy essay (avoid words with the letter *x* or *z*). In the first condition, attention was "depleted." After this task, participants were less able to resist temptation on a test in which it was easy to cheat. Presumably it takes some self-control to resist an easy temptation to cheat. These types of studies suggest that self-control is "domain general"—the same capacity or energy is used to regulate emotion, cognition, action, and impulse—and it behaves as if it depends on some kind of finite resource. They suggest the "resource" can be replenished by rest, and by positive emotion. Controversy has ensued over whether a bit of food replenishes the resource. This has been disproven by comparing results for participants given a bit of sugar water versus allowed to smell some sugar water. Both groups regained capability. It appears that increased motivation (e.g., a signal of a new reward, such as the smell of food) can restore the resource, provided it doesn't create a new distraction. Recent papers have called this phenomenon into question, but these studies provide a useful way to think about the common experience that having to concentrate for a long time can tire us out, some of us more than others.

WANT TO READ MORE?

Mead, N. L., Baumeister, R. F., Gino, F., Schweitzer, M. E., & Ariely, D. (2009). Too tired to tell the truth: Self-control resource depletion and dishonesty. *Journal of Experimental Social Psychology, 45*(3), 594–597.

see it when a child starts to complain unthinkingly before you finish sharing some good news that she will actually like.

> *The capacity to pay attention in the face of distractions is limited, and kids with ADHD have even less than others.*

This also helps us explain why kids with ADHD are often more prone to excessive anxiety or anger—controlling those emotions also takes a certain amount of this limited top-down mental resource. To support that idea, another study by Roy Baumeister's group in 2016 asked high school students to rate their self-control (how well they could deliberately focus, ignore distraction, and follow through on their goals). Five months later they assessed the kids again. Those who rated low on self-control had more test anxiety later on, even after controlling for their earlier test anxiety. While this effect didn't occur for every child, and while other scientists have disputed aspects of this finding, the study is consistent with the idea that the capacity to exert top-down control is closely related to the capacity that helps regulate emotions. When this ability is limited or depleted, trouble with emotion can follow as well.

So to summarize, self-regulation depends on at least three components to work properly:

1. The integrity and efficiency of the "automatic" parts of self-regulation, like detection and filtering of extraneous information, and the brain systems that support those capacities, including the thalamus and the parietal cortex.

2. The integrity and strength of the "top-down" or "deliberate" parts of self-regulation and the brain systems that support those capacities, including the prefrontal cortex, the striatum, and parts of the temporal and parietal cortex and their connections.

 WANT TO READ MORE ABOUT BAUMEISTER'S HIGH SCHOOL SELF-CONTROL STUDY?

Bertrams, A., Baumeister, R. F., & Englert, C. (2016). Higher self-control capacity predicts lower anxiety-impaired cognition during math examinations. *Frontiers of Psychology, 31*(7), 485.

3. The energy or capacity for the top-down or deliberate processes, which depends in part on the noradrenergic system in the brain.

Each of these pieces depends on a different brain system, and there are more systems in addition. But the main idea you should have is that self-regulation includes deliberate or conscious aspects, but also bottom-up or automatic aspects. It's not always the child's effort that is at fault for the fact that she can't self-regulate. *It's not all a matter of willpower.*

Development

IS ADHD JUST A DEVELOPMENTAL DELAY
OR A TRUE DIFFERENCE?

As is obvious to any parent, self-regulation develops remarkably in childhood, while remaining bafflingly limited even in adolescence. In fact, development is nonlinear—that is, in some respects, children have better self-regulation than adolescents. In other respects, adolescents have self-regulation every bit as effective as adults. Science has learned just in the last couple of years that this interesting asymmetric pattern is seen in other species, not just in humans. Development separates self-regulation into different subcapacities. Among these, evolution clearly favors a certain amount of impulsivity and risk taking in the adolescent developmental period for many mammals, including humans.

In some respects, the self-regulation problems of children with ADHD resemble immature behavior. They just seem to regulate more like younger children. Further, some children with ADHD seem to "grow out of" their problems when they become teens or adults. Is ADHD just a delay of normal development? In some respects, and in some cases, it appears to be. For example, a key feature of brain maturation in adolescence is cortical thickness—it peaks in early adolescence and then thins in a particular sequence across the cortex as the brain matures and specializes its many circuits. As a group, teenagers with ADHD show the normal pattern, just about two years later. This may be related to some children "normalizing" their self-regulation as they mature.

However, many other children with ADHD never really catch up. And other aspects of brain development also never quite catch up at the group level. For example, youth with ADHD, as a group, have about 8–10 percent smaller volumes of gray matter in several key brain regions and networks, such as the prefrontal cortex, striatum, and cerebellum. This size reduction seems to emerge early in life and to remain permanent. In this respect, ADHD is not a delay but a different or altered developmental path.

More recently, new brain imaging tools in the past few years have given us the ability to map functional circuits and networks in the brain—to see how the brain has organized its communication system. The communication network in the brain—which parts of the brain talk to other parts—is organized in a particular way, like a telephone network. Just like the old-fashioned phone network had switchboards and modern cellular networks have towers, in the brain some key hubs are connected all over the brain. Other spokes and their nodes are only sparsely interconnected. Work from my colleague Dr. Damien Fair and team in 2015 suggests that the hub, spoke, and node structure appears to be set up differently in typical development, in ADHD, and in autism. This also suggests ADHD is a different form of brain development, not simply a delay in brain maturation.

It may be that within the ADHD group the brains of some children are different in structure and network organization, all resulting in combinations of brain features that enable "recovery" from ADHD and other combinations that prevent "recovery."

Crucially, we have strong reason to believe these brain changes are likely influenced by epigenetic changes, experiences, and learning during the developmental period, as we will see in Chapters 3–8 of this book.

ADHD seems to involve delays in brain development but also differences.

IS ADHD A "DIFFERENCE" OR A "DISABILITY"?

So kids with ADHD have a brain that develops differently. So what? At one level, everyone has unique brain development. Even the patterns of the brain's vascular organization and patterning are unique to each person. Maybe ADHD is just a different way of growing up, not a disorder or a disability. I mentioned that the spontaneous, outgoing, energetic style typical of those with ADHD can be great in some contexts and gives many children with ADHD a delightful quality of "verve" or joie de vivre that no one would want to take away. How boring the world would become if these spirited youngsters were all to quiet down at once!

This question raises deep issues related to culture, the meaning of "illness," and the meaning of "normality," so it rather quickly moves us into the realms of anthropology and philosophy rather than behavioral or clinical science. Suffice to say that the label "disability" can be stigmatizing, disempowering, and harmful—or it can be empowering, beneficial, and organizing. On the harmful side, some scientific studies suggest that in some cases the ADHD label can lead a child to "give up" on himself or lead other children to avoid that child.

The deaf community has developed a subculture that questions whether deafness is something they want to change. Some advocacy groups for those with autism spectrum disorders view autism as a difference from "neurotypical" development, not a disorder. These views have been empowering and strengthening for some individuals with these conditions or developmental pictures.

But let me add to this reflection recent scientific evidence. Several studies have suggested that ADHD is generally not just a disorder, but more like a trait in the population. A medical analogy is blood pressure. When systolic blood pressure is over 140 (or diastolic over 90), we label it as hypertension. This is the case even though a blood pressure of 139 is just one point lower. Blood pressure exists along a continuum. To paraphrase one wag, "Surely the fates love 139 almost as much as 140." There is no magic at 140 instead of 139. But we have to put a cutoff someplace to decide when it's time to intervene medically. Similarly, with ADHD, at a general level most of ADHD is a dimensional trait in the population related to self-regulation. Some people are very disorganized, impulsive, and underregulated. Other people are organized, planful, and well regulated. When the disorganized end of the trait scores 6 or more on our symptom cutoffs, or over 70 on our normative rating scales, we call it a disorder. We do this because as problems get more extreme, we need a decision point at which to say it is time to intervene. With both blood pressure and ADHD, that decision point is simply an actuarial point that seems to provide the best balance between avoiding needless treatment and avoiding neglect of serious risk situations.

How do we know that ADHD is more like a trait? Until recently, the best evidence came from studies of twins. Using mathematical models to compare identical and nonidentical twins, scientists could show that the genetic influences on both normal-range and extreme scores were correlated or the same. Better evidence arrived more recently. Around 2012 or 2013, scientists perfected the mathematical tools, and had enough biological genetic data on enough people, to create biologically based scores for the influence of actual genes on ADHD (and other traits and disorders). These "polygenic risk scores" basically just add up the combined influence of thousands of common gene variants, each having a tiny influence on the outcome. In 2015, these methods were applied for the first time to large samples of people with psychiatric conditions in a worldwide study of thousands of people, and for the first time to ADHD. This analysis, and follow-up studies using those results in 2015 and 2016, confirmed that the same genes had the same level of effect for both normal range and extreme scores on an ADHD measure.

This evidence that the genetic part of the trait is similar at all levels of severity is evidence for a trait, not a separate condition, at the extreme. From this perspective, ADHD is a case of the genetic "volume" (that is, gene expression) turned up too high, placing a child at risk for bad outcomes because she has more, but not different, genetic influences than those with a normal range of this trait.

So far, so good. But now let's turn to the limits on this trait variation viewpoint. The first limit is very practical: even if ADHD is an extreme of a normal trait, the child is still at risk of bad life outcomes—just like someone with high blood pressure. Letting it go as "just a difference" may do a serious disservice to a child who really needs professional help to avoid a very unhappy life. Here the analogy of high blood pressure may have some relevance. The label "ADHD" may also do something good— it may help a family or a teacher to make sense out of a child's struggles. It may guide a clinician on how to help the child. It may help the child see that he's not dumb—rather, he has a condition that requires supports, the way some people need glasses. Clearly, some judgment is necessary to know whether the label will do more harm or more good.

> *Viewing ADHD as simply a difference in a trait may rob individuals of the understanding and treatment they deserve.*

There is a further problem with saying ADHD is just a difference in a trait:

at the group level ADHD is in fact associated with subtle brain injury. For example, low birth weight triples the risk that a child will develop ADHD. It also increases the rate of microscopic ischemic events (loss of blood supply to tissue) that cause damage to certain cells in the brain. Pre- and perinatal loss of blood supply and oxygen from other causes also increases the risk of ADHD. While we don't know whether this is what causes the increase in ADHD in low-birth-weight children or others with more minor complications, it's an obvious possibility. That is, it seems possible, even likely, that at least some children with ADHD have had a subtle injury to their brain that prevented them from reaching their potential. This is not simply normal variation on a trait. It would be a serious disservice to these children to ignore the chance to prevent that injury so that they can reach their full potential.

All of this again underscores the importance of recognizing that children are not all the same: they probably did not all arrive at their difficulties by the same route, and even though they share developmental problems with self-regulation, they probably don't manifest them in the same ways.

In the next chapter, I will explain *epigenetic* and *gene × environment* effects—the major next-generation approach to ADHD. In subsequent chapters, you will learn what we know about modifiable environmental inputs to ADHD—including environmental chemicals, nutritional effects, and stress effects. Anticipating the next chapter, along with what you will learn in Chapters 3–7, enables us to propose a half dozen likely routes to ADHD. You or your child may also be on an "ADHD spectrum" without the full disorder. If, as we now suspect, ADHD is a dimension like blood pressure, then someone who doesn't quite have the full syndrome can still potentially benefit from some of the insights in this book—particularly those ideas that are relatively low risk.

Here are the most likely developmental routes to ADHD, based on current scientific understanding (plus a bit of my own hunches):

1. A simple delay in brain maturation in children who, with the right supports and with time, will develop into "normal range" adults; this could be due to genetic or epigenetic (environmental) influences on development.

2. Normal variation in a common trait (such as over- or underregu-

lation) selected by evolution, which can cause trouble fitting into our modern society; the trait could be moved along the spectrum by an increase or decrease in expression (by analogy, "volume" on the radio dial) on contributing genes, perhaps influenced by epigenetic effects and DNA structure (genotype) in combination.

3. Subtle brain injury interfering with full development of a child's potential, which could be preventable; for example, we know that ADHD is related to several such events, including:

   a. Low birth weight (known since the 1990s).

   b. Extreme parental stress (discovered in the 2000s).

   c. Maternal or paternal exposure to certain environmental chemicals (emerging in the 2000s and 2010s).

   d. Child exposure to certain environmental chemicals (suspected for decades, but clarified and confirmed between 2004 and 2015).

   e. More speculatively, dietary or nutritional insufficiencies (still being studied, but evidence for omega-3 insufficiency associated with ADHD appears strong as of 2015, as discussed later).

4. Genetic mutation interfering with full development of a child's potential, which might benefit from intervention to change gene expression or otherwise compensate for the mutation's biological effects. Here gene expression is driven by the DNA mutation, not epigenetics per se. (Technically, a DNA mutation could change epigenetic expression and cause ADHD, or experiences can change epigenetic expression and cause ADHD.) A few of such rare mutations are known in autism, as shown in a major study in 2016, and we expect to find these for ADHD as well.

5. Known early psychological or biological trauma to the nervous system, including:

   a. Excessive alcohol exposure during pregnancy, causing fetal alcohol syndrome.

   b. Extreme emotional or physical deprivation in early life (e.g., raised in an orphanage with very few staff), causing a particular kind of ADHD condition.

Most of the injuries or stressors described in the preceding list could exert their effects in many ways, but epigenetic change is one likely mechanism, as subsequent chapters will explain. Groups 1 and 2 include children who are developing in the typical range—human variation, which we might speculate was either ignored or selected for during human evolution.

They perhaps just need help fitting into our modern society and as adults need to find the right niche to succeed. However, the other categories include injuries or insults to the developing nervous system that we want to understand, prevent, or compensate for because we value allowing everyone to try to achieve their potential. Failing to prevent or correct an injury, even a subtle one, violates that basic humanistic value.

Most of this book is dedicated to helping you compensate for these setbacks even if you don't know the causal route for your particular child. In fact, generally it is very difficult to identify the route for a particular child because most of you have had children with normal-range environments and only subtle or very common risk inputs. For example, the chemical inputs mentioned above seem to interact with the child's susceptibility, which in turn is partly genetic. I'll explain more about chemicals in Chapter 6.

ADHD: Not a One-Size-Fits-All Condition

If we see ADHD as a problem in self-regulation, most of the seeming contradictions of the disorder come into focus. We can begin to understand the very important variations in how ADHD occurs—through an extreme, or a breakdown, or an alteration, or an injury in one or more of the psychological, cognitive, or biological functions supporting self-regulation. (It's important to understand, however, that ADHD is not the only possible outcome when there is a breakdown in the self-regulation "pipeline"; where the breakdown occurs determines in part whether the outcome is ADHD or obsessive–compulsive disorder or depression, to give just some examples.) We can also begin to grasp the significant variations in how ADHD comes across. In these respects, and with regard to questions about "difference" or "disability," ADHD is not a "one-size-fits-all" condition or label. Fortunately, we can also see that understanding

WHAT'S THE PHYSICAL CAUSE OF SLOW INFORMATION PROCESSING?

Many children with ADHD seem to process and react more slowly than normal when in fast-response situations. The physical basis of this slow processing speed is still unknown. While the brain demands a lot of calories to function, and we know that blood flow increases measurably to certain brain areas when thinking or focusing, and those neurons draw nourishment hungrily, the extra calorie demand for alertness or focused attention is still pretty modest. So it's not just calories, but some other energy route. It may be that a cellular-level energy release mechanism (for example, involving the mitochondria) is involved. It may also be that the glial cells that surround brain cells like insulation are the problem. These glial cells speed up nerve transmission in the brain. There is some evidence that they are underdeveloped in ADHD. This is studied using a special brain imaging technique called diffusion tensor imaging, which shows that the brain's white matter (which might be the glial cells) is not as well developed in kids with ADHD. Related brain imaging using a technique just developed in the last few years looks at the functional connections of brain networks—how well they talk to each other. Here, too, we see a pattern of weaker connections across the brain. This could help explain inefficient "information gain" or processing of information, and thus weak application of controlled attention. Another possibility put forth very recently is a breakdown in the complex energy transmission pipeline from capillaries to neurons that involves cellular glycogen and glucose—a speculation that is as yet untested.

the complexity of self-regulation opens the door to understanding how to help children reach their potential by gaining control over their own actions, emotions, and thoughts. We can do this by supporting how their brain develops. But first, it's important that you see why—that you see the basics of epigenetics.

2

Epigenetics

The End of the
Nature-versus-Nurture Debate

New brain imaging technologies have brought us a new understanding of how the brain develops and how it works. And new genetic discoveries have changed the picture of how ADHD is caused. We no longer view ADHD as a simple matter of the wrong genes, or DNA, causing one part of the brain (like the frontal cortex) to be too small. That model is too simple all the way around. It is far more likely that DNA confers "liability" or "susceptibility" to ADHD. An analogy might be the predisposition to catching a cold. If your child is tired and run down, she will catch a cold at school more easily in the winter. She is more susceptible. Genes can also make us more or less susceptible to a neurodevelopmental problem. The box on the next page describes how scientists know that complex diseases like ADHD are usually related to genetic susceptibility plus other factors.

The emerging insight, likely to become a dominant paradigm in the coming decade, is very different from the old. Where the old paradigm tended to see ADHD, at least implicitly, as basically an inherited condition, the new paradigm sees ADHD as the result of environmental modulation of genetic tendency or susceptibility. We are beginning to see how brain formation, assembly, and development rely on these epigenetic processes.

A major driver of this evolving understanding is a field called *behavioral epigenetics*. *Epigenetics* is a word with many meanings. Some people

FOR COMPLEX DISEASES, GENES CONFER SUSCEPTIBILITY, NOT DISEASE ITSELF

Genetically there are two kinds of disease: simple and complex. Simple disease is caused by a single dominant or recessive gene. Sickle cell anemia is an example of a single-gene recessive disorder. If you get both copies of hemoglobin beta gene on chromosome 11, you get the disease. PKU (phenylketonuria) is a single-gene neurodevelopmental disorder. Kids with PKU get the disease if they get two copies of the PAH gene on chromosome 12. Complex disease is caused by a combination of factors—either two or more genes, or a partially expressed gene in which a gene's expression is modified by other factors, or a gene or genes plus an environmental trigger. A complex disease can also include some cases caused by a single major genetic mutation, but that mutation does not explain most of the disease, only isolated cases. Most modern diseases are complex diseases—these include cancer, diabetes, obesity, and psychiatric disorders. Even infectious disease is complex, because it combines genetic susceptibility (usually conveyed by a combination of several genes) with an infectious microbe. For example, a major review of twin studies of tuberculosis revealed that tuberculosis had a twin heritability similar to that of ADHD. That means the susceptibility variation in the population is mostly genetic. However, tuberculosis obviously is present only when an infection follows. In an analogous way, ADHD is probably caused not by DNA, but by DNA-transmitted susceptibility, combined with particular environments. In a study my colleagues and I published in 2016, we demonstrated this "proof of concept" using the environmental pollutant lead (see Chapter 6 for more on lead). We showed that the association between supposedly mild levels of lead exposure and ADHD was quite strong or quite weak depending on which mutation of the HFE gene a child had. The HFE gene modulates iron uptake in the gut; iron in turn interacts with lead to change the final metabolic effect on the brain.

have used it simply to mean the vast array of developmental changes "on top of" the genome that occur during development. But I intend a specific biological meaning. That meaning refers to specific stable biological changes in which the body forms a chemical marker to attach to the DNA molecule, changing its expression in a particular cell or type of cell. That change is sustained over time (e.g., during cell division) and sometimes inherited across human generations. This definition is consistent with the current definition used by the U.S. National Institutes of Health.

This change in gene expression influences behavior and health. Types of epigenetic changes include DNA methylation, micro-RNA expression, and histone modification, among others. Let's take DNA methylation, the most common type of epigenetic change, as an example. A molecule called a methyl group attaches to the DNA, blocking that particular DNA molecule from RNA transcription—in effect, "turning off" the gene in that cell. This changes the RNA signature and the chemical cascade and biological effects of the gene—including in the brain. Removing the methyl group molecule can turn the gene back on. Some epigenetic changes are preprogrammed in our DNA (like the differentiation of cells into neurons, skins cells, and so on during development). They can also be caused by random changes (just as genetic mutations can occur randomly). However, significant epigenetic change can also be caused by experiences. In this way our experiences literally "get under our skin" and are remembered in our biology. That is our focus here, because it opens up new ways that ADHD can be affected by changing a child's experience or environment.

Therefore, whether a disease or a disorder like ADHD actually develops depends on two things: (1) DNA-transmitted susceptibility and (2) environmentally modulated gene expression or regulation. The gene regulation depends on numerous factors, including other DNA elsewhere in a person's genome, as well as different kinds of epigenetic effects, of which DNA methylation is one. Epigenetic changes like DNA methylation can be caused by both biological and psychological experiences, including nutrition, pollution exposure, stress, learning, and others discussed in the rest of this book.

We can say with confidence that genes don't determine who you are; rather genes in interplay with the environment shape our development. In a statistical analysis, this interaction of DNA and experience is called *genotype × environment interaction* or G×E. You'll see a lot of studies on G×E if you venture into the medical or psychological literature these days. One way G×E carries out its effects is by epigenetic change. Epigenetic change is to DNA as control dials are to the electronic circuits on your car stereo. The stereo plays something very different when you change the bass–treble ratio, change the volume, or even change the station. After you change the settings, the new volume stays that way until you change the dial again. Yet the underlying electronics have not changed. Similarly, an epigenetic change happens on a gene in response to an event and then remains there, on the DNA, for a period of time until something happens to reverse it. The original epigenetic change may have been due to an event—say a very stressful pregnancy, or exposure to pesticides in the home, or lead in the school, or eating a very healthy or very unhealthy diet. The change then has a certain stability. Just like the radio volume doesn't change until something happens (you turn the dial again), the gene expression altered by the epigenetic mark after an experience may stay that way until another event reverses it or adds to it. For example, it appears that the epigenetic changes caused by stress can be reversed by aerobic exercise (see Chapters 4 and 7).

It is likely that most complex diseases and behaviors related to conditions like ADHD are related to GxE. We call it GxE because the same epigenetic change doesn't happen to everyone who has a particular exposure or experience. The effect is an interplay between the experience and the person's other characteristics, including the individual's DNA.

How Did We Get Here?

Historically, two major—and oversimplified—theories about what causes ADHD and about how people develop self-control or self-regulation have pervaded our society. The first says that it's all about the parents. If you were a better parent, your child would behave better! Some of you probably believe this about yourself, and you blame yourself for your child's ADHD problems. I have worked with parents who are quite depressed because they are sure their child's ADHD is due to their inability to parent effectively. The second basic explanation is that it's genetic. This idea took over in the 1980s and 1990s as genetic research got under way and studies of identical twins showed not only that ADHD runs in families but also that most of the variation between people is due to variation in their genes. This led some professionals and parents to think that the only way to treat ADHD is biologically (medication) and that a person with ADHD is fated to have it for life—after all, it's genetic, and things that are genetic supposedly never change!

Researchers studying stigma find that families with ADHD get unfairly stigmatized either way. While some of this rejection is related to reactions to the child's difficult behavior, other reactions seem to be based on stereotypes of what ADHD is. Parents are shunned sometimes because other parents don't want "failed parents" (as they mistakenly see it) and their "badly raised" kids around. But when people believe ADHD is genetic, they see the child with ADHD as defective and still don't want to be close to her or the family.

The most recent science has enabled an increasingly clear alternative understanding. We can now see that while both ideas (early experience and genetics as cause of ADHD) have a truth to teach us, both are so oversimplified as to be more misleading than useful by themselves. The new and coming science of ADHD and of human development is teaching us a new way to understand genetics, while also showing us much more about how parents can help their children develop self-control, self-regulation, and healthy maturity.

The End of the Naive Genetic Paradigm

We know that ADHD runs in families and that genetic variation accounts for a lot of that, from twin studies. In fact, the past thirty years have been eye-opening in demonstrating the widespread influence of genetic makeup on nearly all aspects of human variation, from personality to intellectual ability. But genotype is far from the entire story. The simplistic genetic paradigm for ADHD (and other diseases, traits, and behaviors) was that genetics is genetics is genetics: Just like you can inherit blue eyes or Huntington's disease from your parents, you inherit ADHD. And if you do, well, according to this simplistic view, that's just bad luck. Not much you can do about it (at least at our present level of technology; see the box on the next page for a peek into the future). DNA indeed doesn't change after conception. Many experts not too long ago believed it was just a matter of time before we discovered the major gene or genes responsible for ADHD.

GENE EDITING

Scientists have developed many ways to turn genes on and off, but most of these are complex, difficult, and costly, and often not as precise as needed to treat human disease. Changing methylation is one very exciting new direction, as illustrated in examples in the text. But work has also continued on editing genes (splicing). Gene editing has typically required using custom proteins (called restriction enzymes) that can cut a gene and splice it. These techniques have been used to create genetically modified crops and to cure mice of a genetic disease in the lab. But genetic therapies for humans have remained at a very primitive stage due to the lack of precision control in this method. A simpler method has now taken the scientific world by storm, called CRISPR-Cas9. It is based on the discovery in 2012 and 2013 that certain bacteria already do gene editing very precisely (perhaps developed in evolution as a way to fight viruses). In 2015, a nonviable human embryo was genetically modified (then destroyed), provoking calls for a ban on human embryo editing due to the unresolved bioethical issues. CRISPR-Cas allows microsurgery on exactly the portion of the gene of interest. Now instead of just turning a gene's volume up or down, scientists have the potential to "change the station"—to change what the gene produces. In the future, it may be possible to edit the gene that causes single-gene disorders like Huntington's disease and cure or prevent the disease. It is still not clear how far this technology can go to address complex diseases like mental or neurodevelopmental disorders by removing the associated genetic liability and thus preventing them, but that science fiction scenario, while not likely to occur in our lifetime, still has come one step closer to reality.

WANT TO LEARN MORE ABOUT GENE EDITING?

For explanations accessible to the layperson, see the August 2016 issue of *National Geographic* (*www.nationalgeographic.com/magazine/2016/08/dna-crispr-gene-editing-science-ethics*) or watch the TED Talk by Dr. Jennifer Doudna, who made the initial discovery in 2012 (*www.youtube.com/watch?v=TdBAHexVYzc*).

While it is true that there's a substantial genetic influence on ADHD, this simplistic idea of what genetics means is now outdated. The paradigm has turned out to be wrong in two major ways:

1. There is no single gene (or even a few genes) responsible for causing ADHD.

2. What is inherited via DNA is not ADHD itself—it is a propensity.

Twenty years of research have failed to find "the gene" for ADHD or any other major behavior or mental disorder. Scientists now recognize that this is because, with the exception of some rare genetic mutations that occur in only a small number of cases, most of ADHD is influenced not by one major gene but by hundreds or thousands of tiny genetic effects. As this book goes to press the Psychiatric Genetics Consortium is preparing to report genetic results from a study of over 20,000 ADHD cases and 35,000 controls from twelve sites around the world (although more than 14,000 of the cases and 20,000 controls are from Denmark). Results reveal the first confirmation of genetic markers that are statistically dependable in ADHD—but each marker has only a small effect. While we are now beginning to identify these individual effects, the large number of small effects means that genes aren't destiny; rather, they affect probability. An old slogan of medieval soothsayers was purported to be "The stars incline but do not compel"; a similar logic is about right for how genes work in complex disease and human traits.

Second, mathematical proofs show that the twin studies reveal not that we inherit ADHD but that we inherit what genetic scientists call *liability* to disease or outcome. A commonsense proof of this came from twin studies of infectious diseases like tuberculosis, which also show substantial heritability of liability. While ADHD does not result from infectious disease, the concept is analogous. This liability may either be a vulnerability (at risk for ADHD with no compensating benefit) or a susceptibility (extra-sensitive to environmental inputs for good or for ill). To put it simply, complex diseases and disorders like ADHD are rarely if ever caused by genes on their own, but typically by specific sets of genes in the context of specific developmental experiences. These experiences act like triggers that bring to fruition the potential in the genes.

> *We don't inherit ADHD. We inherit a propensity, liability, susceptibility, or sensitivity to developing it.*

This makes sense if you reflect on it—when someone comes to work sick, not everyone gets sick even though everyone was exposed. Part of the reason is inevitably genetic differences in our propensity to catch colds. But on the other hand, the genetic propensity to catch a cold won't guarantee you catch a cold—if you avoid exposure, wash your hands, and are well nourished, you may avoid most colds even though you are genetically vulnerable. Vulnerability itself is a combination of genetic propensity, environmental risk and protection, and a particular disease-triggering exposure.

In the past decade, and particularly in the past five years, these genotype × environment combinations have moved from concepts into proven specifics. Scientists now have discovered specific G×E interactions related to child behavior and emotional problems, learning problems, and neural development. Several G×E effects are now established in mental disorders. See the box on page 47 for a couple of examples.

The genes discussed in the box are also suspected or known to be associated with ADHD. For example, my colleagues and I and another group of researchers independently reported in 2016 that ADHD is associated with mutations on the serotonin transporter promoter gene interacting with parenting characteristics. Other genes may have similar interaction effects with the social or biological environment but are not yet confirmed. (I will discuss some other very important G×E effects in later chapters.) Although the specific effects in ADHD are not as robustly established to date as the effects in depression (a handful of studies versus the eighty-one studies to date in depression), the direction is clear: G×E interactions are increasingly seen as involved in the development of ADHD.

It is crucial to remember, as also noted in the box, that these G×E effects may sometimes involve not just increased risk for disease or for ADHD (what some scientists specify as genetic vulnerability) but rather increased *sensitivity to experience* (what some scientists specify as the meaning of genetic susceptibility). In other words, it may not be accurate to say that some children are prone to ADHD and others are not. It may be more accurate to say that some

> Rather than saying that G×E makes some children more likely to have ADHD, it may be more accurate to say that G×E makes some of them more sensitive to early life experiences.

EXAMPLES OF RECENTLY DISCOVERED GxE INTERACTIONS IN MENTAL HEALTH

Depression. A 2016 review of the literature noted that stressful life events (in utero or in childhood) are more likely to result in depression for children later if they have particular alleles (mutations) of one of a handful of genes that affect brain signaling in the frontal cortex and other brain regions. The most well established is the serotonin transporter gene. The association of depression with the interaction of mutations on that gene and stressful events was confirmed in a formal meta-analysis of eighty-one studies reported in 2014. The probability that this GxE interaction is a chance effect is less than one in 1 million. Other studies suggest that these GxE effects on depression are transmitted by epigenetic changes in susceptible individuals.

Antisocial Behavior. The monoamine oxidase type-A brain receptor has a particular gene that encodes it, called the MAO-A brain receptor gene. It has a promoter polymorphism that confers susceptibility to aggression and antisocial behavior. Children in an antisocial peer group or exposed to abuse were seen in several studies to be more likely to develop aggressive and antisocial behavior when they had this particular gene mutation. This effect was supported by findings in a large national study in 2016, where children exposed to physical abuse were found to be more likely to become aggressive and antisocial if they had this gene mutation. However, most intriguing was evidence from another large study in 2016. There, one particular MAO-A marker along with another genetic mutation, called COMT, interacted with parenting styles—"for good and for ill." That is, children with the sensitive genotypes were more likely to be aggressive when they had too little positive parenting and more likely to be prosocial when they had enough positive parenting.

INTERESTED IN READING MORE?

Sharma, S., et al. (2016). Gene × environment determinants of stress- and anxiety-related disorders. *Annual Review of Psychology, 67,* 216–239.

Sharpley, C. F., Palanisamy, S. K., Glyde, N. S., Dillingham, P. W., & Agnew, L. L. (2014). An update on the interaction between the serotonin transporter promoter variant (5-HTTLPR), stress and depression, plus an exploration of non-confirming findings. *Behavioral Brain Research, 273*(15), 89–105. Note that important variation in results of these studies suggest that other genes or experiences may over-ride these effects or create subtypes of depression.

Lu, Y. F., & Menard, S. (2017). The interplay of MAOA and peer influences in predicting adult criminal behavior. *Psychiatric Quarterly, 88*(1), 115–128.

WANT TO READ MORE ABOUT G×E ASSOCIATION BETWEEN ADHD AND PARENTING?

Elmore, A. L., Nigg, J. T., Friderici, K. H., & Nikolas, M. A. (2016). Does 5HTTLPR genotype moderate the association of family environment with child attention-deficit hyperactivity disorder symptomatology? *Journal of Clinical Child and Adolescent Psychology, 45*(3), 348–360.

Morgan et al. (2016). Parental serotonin transporter polymorphism (5-HTTLPR) moderates associations of stress and child behavior with parenting behavior. *Journal of Clinical Child and Adolescent Psychology, 18*, 1–12.

children are exceptionally sensitive or responsive to their early experiences, for good or for ill, compared to others. Based on current evidence, it is likely that both effects influence child development, but it is too early to tell how much each kind of effect bears on ADHD.

As I note again later in the book, some gene × environment interactions are very important for another reason. They may show us how a particular genotype in a child indicates a need for a particular intervention—a particular change in a nutrient, for example. Genetic research is also very important for showing us what kinds of physiological systems are driving some aspects of ADHD, and this can open up new treatment ideas for influencing those systems. For example, if inflammation is involved, then treatments to reduce inflammation may be helpful.

Can a G×E interaction cause a change in the brain and behavior? If so, how? The answer to both questions comes from recent studies that directly examined epigenetics.

How Powerful a Role Does Epigenetics Play?

Scientifically, when basic chemical compounds attach to the DNA in response to an experience, they change which genes are expressed and by how much. These epigenetic effects can be quite powerful—just as large as genetic effects. In a sense, they can seem to override genetic effects. For example, in a classic experiment at Duke in 2007, Randy Jirtle and his colleagues cloned genetically identical agouti mice (essentially identical twins) and had them carried to term by two different genetically identical mothers. The mothers lived in identical conditions except that one group was exposed to bisphenol A (BPA), a plastic chemical found at that time in many food containers (discussed more in Chapter 6). After birth, the genetically identical animals had identical rearing conditions and identical diets and chemical exposures. Yet the group exposed to BPA was large, fat, and yellow, and the other group small, lean, and brown. The first group had a change in DNA methylation that caused the agouti gene (and other genes) to express differently and create this difference in their growth. They also had behavioral differences. They were more different, by virtue of this early chemical exposure, than two genetically different strains of mouse. Those events occurred in skin (causing pigment changes) and in the brain (causing changes in feeding behavior and satiety and leading to obesity).

During pregnancy, such negative epigenetic effects can be prevented by counteracting the effects of the environment. Proof of this concept emerged when Jirtle and colleagues also showed in 2007 that certain dietary supplements during pregnancy, such as folic acid and vitamin B_{12}, were sufficient to prevent these epigenetic marks from being created by the BPA. These types of supplements provided additional methyl molecules that make up for the methylation lost from the BPA exposure. The supplementation also reduced disease incidence later, even in the mice not exposed to BPA.

Since then, data have rapidly accumulated regarding the positive and negative epigenetic changes caused by different environments, both in utero and during childhood. While most of the work is in animals, parallel effects are also now being seen in humans. (We are much harder to study because it is difficult to get to epigenetic change in our brains, so scientists have to rely on indirect evidence from human saliva or blood, combined with direct studies of brains in animals and, rarely, a postmortem study.) In later chapters you'll see how even as children are growing up, positive epigenetic change can occur, and negative epigenetic change can be reversed, by factors like exercise and nutrition. Negative epigenetic changes can be avoided by avoiding experiences like exposure to chemicals such as BPA. While showing these effects in animals is not the same as showing them in humans, it is highly suggestive, and some converging human evidence is beginning to emerge.

Why would a different experience, like exercise or diet, counteract the effects of stress or chemical exposure? One emerging model suggests that numerous early "insults" to development work through changes in a complex hormonal network involving inflammation, corticosteroid hormones, oxidative stress, and related processes that may be shared across numerous challenges—from poor diet to chemical exposure, to sustained emotional stress or trauma. Thus, as we learn more about how gene and environment effects work on those internal communication systems, we begin to see the outlines of a developmental process that can sidetrack brain development—and also provide tools for helping it get back on track.

The epigenetic changes caused by exposure to some environmental factors may be counteracted by exposure to a different environmental factor—dietary supplements during pregnancy protecting against exposure to certain toxic chemicals, exercise protecting against the effects of stress, and more. Such findings hold exciting possibilities for preventing or treating ADHD.

Fortunately, a great many of the chemical responses to experience via epigenetics are *conserved* across species. This means that when we do look across species, we can see the same chemical events happening, and the same ones affecting the brain. We need only a few confirmations of this principle of conservation to use the animal findings. Even though human behavior has more determinants than animal behavior (such as our imagination of the future), if we have some of these confirmations already in hand, we can get a long way on what we know.

The fact that many of the same chemical effects on the brain occur from species to species means that animal studies offer us a wealth of interventions to explore.

 WANT TO READ MORE ABOUT DIETARY SUPPLEMENTS PROTECTING AGAINST BPA EXPOSURE DURING PREGNANCY?

Dolinov, D. C., Huang, D., & Jirtle, R. L. (2007). Maternal nutrient supplementation counteracts bisphenol A-induced DNA hypomethylation in early development. *Proceedings of the National Academy of Science, 104*(32), 13056–13061.

We don't actually know how much of ADHD's heritability is epigenetic rather than genetic, but my bet is that it will prove to be substantial. I believe that ADHD is not fated from conception and that there's a lot of hope for correcting it. We just need to learn how. The view I suggest is that ADHD becomes more or less likely at conception due to genetic makeup. But its expression can and does change in relation to early and later development both in the womb and throughout childhood and adolescence.

Can Epigenetics Exert Their Influence across Generations?

The bottom line here is that epigenetic change can occur both before birth and during childhood (and maybe during adulthood). These changes can be positive or negative for health. They are fairly stable, but many if not all can be reversed by further experiences of the right type. It remains unknown to what extent the undoing of these effects must occur by a certain age. For example, we don't yet know to what extent epigenetic changes stabilize after early childhood. However, animal studies show that at least some epigenetic effects can be reversed by experiences well into later childhood or early adult development and perhaps beyond. In later chapters, I particularly highlight low-risk, healthy steps that also have some evidence of either protecting against or reversing epigenetic harm. In addition, making the effort to reverse negative changes can be beneficial to your child, and it may even prove beneficial for your grandchildren. That's because in some cases, if they are not reversed, epigenetic changes are passed on to the next generation. They can be in the "germ line" that passes on through the egg or sperm to an individual's offspring. In effect they "ride along" on the DNA in inheritance. The DNA brings with it a chemical memory of some of the parents' experiences (both fathers' and mothers') and passes it to the child.

Epigenetic change has the power to affect not only your child's life but the lives of future generations, as these changes ride along on the child's DNA.

The genetic inputs to ADHD therefore are an important part of the puzzle and remain a fascinating and important area of study. In fact, my laboratory is heavily invested in studying DNA changes associated with ADHD to help us understand biological systems in ADHD as well as genetic vulnerability and susceptibility. It is a virtual certainty that exciting findings will emerge from worldwide genetic studies going forward. But these will probably shed light on liability to ADHD and need to be completed by understanding the role of the environment. Therefore, my lab is also heavily invested in studying epigenetic effects associated with ADHD. Because epigenetic changes coming from early and subsequent experiences probably carry so much potential for new treatments and for insights you can use in your daily life, this book focuses mainly on the wealth of new discoveries about how experience changes the genome, the brain, and behavior and development, how we can apply that to ADHD now—and how we might do so even more in the future.

What Does This All Mean for the Brain?

The past generation has filled in many of the blanks in the truly astonishing processes of brain development. We now know, for example, that the brain develops dramatically not just before birth and during infancy, but all the way until the mid-twenties—especially the aspects of the brain necessary for mature self-regulation. This development includes not only growth but also pruning that hones the brain's ability to meet ever-growing cognitive demands ever more efficiently:

- Very early life sees the "build-out" of neurons and neural connections, with a peak of neural connections at about age two. This neural "overgrowth" is what gives the human brain its remarkable versatility during infancy and toddlerhood. You have probably heard that a one-year-old can effortlessly learn any language in the world perfectly just by living with it, and you're probably well aware that this is no longer possible for you as an adult.

- Beginning around the toddler years, the brain begins a long process of specialization by pruning less-used or ineffective neural patterns and solidifying those that are used and that work well to make us more efficient. This is how the child specializes for the niche, culture, or situation she is in.

- Development also includes the expansion of myelin, the coating around neural axons (connecting wires) that gives them their transmission speed—it gives them the equivalent of an upgrade from copper wire to fiber optics in terms of capacity and speed of information. This upgrade continues all the way into early adulthood.

- This build-out of the communication wires goes on through the first two or more decades of life. During adolescence, certain parts of the brain peak in size and begin to shrink to become maximally efficient.

- Also during adolescence, the brain is set up to lower the intensity of signals about risky situations—encouraging the adolescent to explore the world and take chances doing so. This pattern is seen not just in humans but in other mammals as well. That's part of the reason adolescents can seem so impulsive while at other times being so reflective.

- Finally, neural networks communicate and solidify their relationships through frequent "oscillations" of shared electrochemical activity, in which they get familiar with their mutual firing patterns and develop practiced skill routines for adaptation to adult life. Basically, they establish a channel of regular communication so that when brain region A fires, region B pays attention—region A's signals have been useful before and so are probably useful now too. This is how the brain learns, for example, to get a handle on strong emotions—region B (in the frontal cortex) learns to fire at the same time as region A (in another part of the brain) to modulate a signal of excitement or fear.

We also know that all of these major developmental processes are influenced by four major factors:

1. Genetic signals

2. Prenatal environment signals, mostly via food and maternal hormones such as stress hormones, but also via chemical exposures, all of which involve epigenetic signals

3. Ongoing childhood learning, experience, or stress, with its own epigenetic recordings

4. Adversity, trauma, or subtle injury throughout one's life but especially during childhood development

Because of the role of experience and learning and its epigenetic recording in governing brain sculpting, human brain development is very sensitive, or responsive to its environment. That environment includes learning, experience, and stress, as well as food, chemical toxicants, and all physical and social inputs.

The main goal of this book is to explain the small set of critically important influences on the health of the developing brain and how you might harness those influences to counteract a genetic predisposition to ADHD, to minimize its severity in a child already diagnosed, or even to reduce heritability in future generations.

Where Are We Headed?

The naive genetic paradigm is done, just as the naive environmental paradigm before it. We need genetics to understand susceptibility and vulnerability. But ADHD is best seen as coming from the interplay of genetic and environmental susceptibility and environmental triggers. Increasingly, this concept is moving away from a bland, generic "all of the above" assertion to very specific proposals regarding particular environments (and associated particular genes) and their differential relation to ADHD and overlapping conditions. This line of work converges with animal and human studies of specific environments to overturn some common beliefs from before. Chemical exposures were once dismissed as an unimportant influence on ADHD; that's no longer accurate. Similarly, both prenatal and childhood diet was thought to be unimportant. That is now changing. The long-standing neglect of the role of social disadvantage, trauma, and stress on ADHD (or ADHD-like problems) is also being corrected. The size of all these effects is not necessarily as big as some advocates would have you believe—but it's still meaningful and on occasion can be decisive. My purpose is to help you get the right balance and understanding, to see the exciting possibilities, yet use them in a level-headed way, and to help you judge what will work for your particular situation. I hope by the end of this book you'll see that in addition to professional help, you have a lot of options for helping your child—enough that you can choose the ones that will be both beneficial for your child and manageable for you and your family. Here are a couple of examples:

When Addison came in for his ADHD evaluation at age eight, he was irritable, short-tempered, inattentive, and restless. His parents noted that even though he could have a lot of fun playing, when left with nothing to do he just couldn't seem to settle down. After consulting with friends, their pediatrician, and other sources, they began to consider food as one option. It dawned on them that he also was a picky eater and had consistent digestion problems such as constipation. They got advice from a dietician and undertook several key diet changes discussed in Chapter 3. Gradually, after several months, Addison began to be calmer, less irritable, more focused. He also enjoyed his food more, was hungrier, and had better digestion. While it's not always the case that food-related problems and ADHD come with obvious digestive issues, and while dietary changes may help only a minority of children with ADHD, the pattern here was notable and consistent with what new studies have shown can happen.

Machiko, by age eight, was having frequent arguments and fights with other children, was losing friends because she was too bossy, and had frequent temper tantrums at home that her single mother, Tori, described as "drama-queen" overreactions. Machiko had been diagnosed with ADHD in first grade due to her restlessness, overactivity, and inability to focus for any length of time on her schoolwork. She had been started on a medication, but the effects were not very clear. Consulting with her nurse practitioner, Tori acknowledged that their life had been difficult for a long time. When Machiko was a preschooler, Tori's boyfriend was physically abusive to Tori, which Machiko witnessed. The subsequent moves, first to Tori's parents and then out to an apartment, had been disruptive. Machiko also didn't seem to sleep very well. The nurse practitioner had read that consistent exercise can help reverse some of the effects of emotional trauma. Tori thought exercise would be good for her own trauma as well. After changing her work schedule, she arranged for Machiko to take a long bike ride with her after school every day. On days when the weather was bad, they went to the gym together and competed to see who could do the most stairs on the StairMaster machine. While Machiko didn't like this at first, Tori was able to motivate her with points for how far they rode or how many stairs climbed and make it into a game they did together. After several weeks the habits took hold and the routine was in place, and after a few months Tori noticed that Machiko was having fewer blowups and tantrums. She finished third grade, and fourth grade became a much easier year. Machiko was sleeping better, was less hyperactive, paying better attention, and now seemed to get a full benefit from the medication, which she could now take at a lower dosage. While exercise won't always have major effects, it can reverse some epigenetic effects of trauma and also help grow the brain's "executive function" networks that help with self-regulation. The experience of Tori and Machiko, while certainly not universal, is consistent with what the literature says can happen. There is average benefit shown in the science—which likely conceals larger benefits for some children. A bonus was that Machiko's improved sleep was part of a virtuous cycle that had begun to replace the vicious cycle of bad days and bad sleep.

And there are more exciting possibilities on the horizon for helping children with ADHD or overall self-regulation problems. In the coming years, genetic studies will be used to understand how experience and genes work together in specific ways in large biological systems. Epigenetic tools will become important. ADHD will be one of the puzzles we'll understand. This information in turn will tell us how to modify the genetic effect to treat or cure disease or disorder and help kids reach their potential. This won't all be possible with today's tools—it will take new tools, to be invented in the future, perhaps even the far future. But we can take advantage of this insight now with a fresh understanding of how the environment, including everyday events, shapes epigenetic change, brain development, and growth in children. You'll read what we currently know about low-tech approaches to improving ADHD symptoms in the next five chapters.

3

Food and ADHD

Old Controversies and New Clarity

In Chapter 2 we noted that the brain develops dramatically and is exquisitely dependent on and responsive to its early developmental circumstances. Nutrition is therefore important for everyone—but if your child
has ADHD, you likely have less margin for error as a parent and want to
know whether you should go the extra mile. It's probably hard to determine because one of the biggest and most passionate historical controversies about ADHD has been whether diet can cause it or help it. Further, food becomes a fad—almost religious in fervor—for some people.
The bottom line for ADHD is that in just the last five years, the scientific
view on this has changed from "No—diet is just a fad and cannot affect
ADHD" to "Wait, maybe it can." While quite a few limits remain on that
claim, we've got enough here to send you in the right direction and sort
the wheat from the chaff.

Most notable is that state-of-the art meta-analytic findings in 2012,
2013, and 2014 established two points:

- Omega-3 (fish oil) supplementation can help ADHD.

- Food additives and allergens affect some children in ways that can
  mimic ADHD—and in some cases their removal can help with
  ADHD.

The second conclusion may seem like old news—but it still surprises many parents to find out that added sugar, for all its other devastating effects on child health, is not a main cause of inattention. It is more likely the other additives in sugary food that trigger reactions in some children. The remaining controversies about diet pertain to how many children with ADHD have diet as a component of the disorder, how to predict ahead of time which children would respond to a diet-based change, and how big the benefits of trying a diet change might be.

Meanwhile, provided your child shows no signs of deficiency in iron, zinc, or vitamin D, the jury is out on the value of other single-nutrient or multinutrient supplements. Multinutrient and mega-nutrient vitamin and mineral supplements, however, are an area of active investigation in ADHD. They may ultimately prove to help almost as much as a more comprehensive diet change. New insights into the role of inflammation in disease and the importance of the "gut–brain axis" have fueled specu- lation that neurodevelopmental disorders like ADHD are related to an inflammatory digestive reaction from food. This has resulted in interest in anti-inflammatory foods, probiotic supplements, and other new ideas. This chapter will update you on what we do—and don't—yet know about their value as well. Further, it is increasingly clear that maternal diet, as well as possibly obesity during pregnancy, is important to child behavior and may affect ADHD. I'll get you up to speed here too.

Overall, while we await consensus on all these secondary points, enough new findings have crystallized in recent years that it's time for a fresh look at the opportunities to help your child with ADHD through diet.

The context here bothers some parents. We live in a strangely dual world. Many children are still undernourished—even in the United States. Around the world over 600 million people and a third of all schools lack safe drinking water and over 2 billion people (30 percent of the planet) lack sanitary toilets. Every twenty seconds a child dies due to poor sanitation; over 100 million children suffer stunted growth from starvation. Yet the noncommunicable diseases traditionally associated with the first world—obesity, diabetes, heart disease, cancer, and mental illnesses like schizophrenia, depression, ADHD, and autism—are rapidly becoming the main health-related source of suffering everywhere. Food is part of the problem. In the first world, many people are "overnour-ished"—or getting too many "empty calories" with lots of food but not enough nutrition. Our food is often processed in ways that add nonfood chemicals (often to preserve the food or make it look more appetizing). The processing at one level is understandable—it means we can get food from all over the world cheaply. That leaves us more money to pay the rent. But it comes at a high cost to health.

The relevant news for ADHD is that many of the food problems that contribute to health issues like obesity and diabetes also interfere with brain development. In other words, the good news, if I can put it that way, is that you can support your child's brain health and her physi-cal health through the *same* dietary considerations. A few key steps are relevant to ADHD.

The challenge for parents, for all of us, is simply finding healthy food for our children. Too often school lunches are loaded with added sugar or processed food with additives. At the grocery store, the lower-cost food is often the most processed and least healthy. Fresh and organic food, free of additives or pesticide residue, often costs more. You are all familiar with trying to cut through the myriad, and seemingly changeable, dietary recommendations that bombard us all. More fat? More protein? Supple-ments? Let's sort it out.

The bottom line: A sea change is under way. Unlike in the past, if you think your child's ADHD may have something to do with food, science now agrees with you.

I'll quickly review the latest science on food and the brain, including a reminder about dietary health "basics" that many readers may already be familiar with. Then I'll move on to the latest science on effective, as well as claimed but unproven, dietary strategies for ADHD. I've orga-nized these roughly from simplest to most difficult, so as you think about your own level of ambition in addressing dietary or nutritional health for your child with ADHD you can step in at the level appropriate to your situation.

While many other scientists and I were long skeptical of the role of food in ADHD, new and better studies just in the period from 2011 to 2015 have changed the landscape. We now have scientific evidence for these statements:

- Food additives, food allergens, and food nutrients, particularly proper fat ratios, broadly influence attention, temperament, and behavior in children.

- Prenatal diet is important to children's subsequent temperament and brain growth.

- Changing diet *can* sometimes cause improvement in ADHD symptoms.

- Omega-3 supplementation is a reliable way to reduce ADHD symptoms, although not as much as standard treatments.

- These benefits, although *small on average,* can be significant for some children.

Exactly how many children with ADHD would benefit from some type of dietary change remains unclear. What is clear is that looking closely at your child's "fuel"—food—offers you an opportunity to promote your child's brain growth and self-regulation and improve ADHD-related problems.

Food's Importance to Brain Health: What the Science Tells Us

The importance of food to brain health and functioning has been underscored in astonishing fashion in the past few years with the discovery of the *microbiome* and its relation to the communication channel called the gut–brain axis. We now know that the gut is connected to the brain via a complex set of nerves. This pathway includes brain chemicals, or neurotransmitters. It turns out that the gut also contains some of these brain chemicals. The gut–brain axis depends on the microbiome, or microbes in the gut. There are many types of these microbes, one of which is called *probiotic*. That discovery has spurred a recent craze for "probiotic supplements" among health-food enthusiasts.

> *Over half of the DNA and cells in the human body are not human but bacterial. These microbes, called the microbiome, are essential to digestion as well as to brain health.*

Scientists now study the human microbiome to understand its role in health and development. These microscopic organisms live all over our body, but most are in the digestive tract. A recent, striking discovery is that the human body contains more bacterial DNA than human DNA, and more bacterial than human cells! (It's also emerging that we have a lot of friendly viruses as well, but we know more about bacteria, so I talk only about those here.)

Friendly bacteria cover us and live throughout our body, helping us thrive in this specific environment called earth, in which we evolved. They and we have evolved together as a symbiotic co-organism over millions of years. Were it not for the bacteria, we would not be here. Were it not for us, they would not have taken anything like their current form. We cannot live without them, and they cannot live without us. They do everything from help us digest food to send signals to the rest of the body to guide energy allocation.

The gut and the brain "talk to each other" via specific nerve pathways that are only now being understood, including the vagus system (long of interest in its own right to scientists who study self-regulation and ADHD), the enteric nervous system, the endocrine system (which is related to stress response as well as other functions), and the immune system. To put it somewhat metaphorically, inflammation triggered in the gut can "travel" to the brain and affect brain function. That in turn affects mood, attention, and behavior.

The most convincing research on the relevance of the gut to the brain and behavior has emerged just since 2004 in animal experiments and mostly on animal behaviors that mimic human anxiety or mood. It seems almost certain that similar effects will hold for attention and other behaviors. While the microbiome is a current "hot topic," and therefore can be oversold, it nonetheless helps us understand just how vital diet and nutrition are to brain health.

It is important to note that brain growth and health don't depend on the microbiome alone. Brain activity relies heavily on the macronutrients of fat, especially the long-chain fatty acids called omega-3s, carbohydrates, and proteins (amino acids). It also relies on vitamin and mineral micronutrients such as iron, zinc, and calcium, which are crucial to neural transmission and brain health.

Diet during Pregnancy and Early Childhood: How Food May Change the Risk of ADHD and What You Can Do about It

Diet can affect brain growth directly by supplying (or not supplying) necessary nutrients. But nutrients also alter development by triggering epigenetic changes, both during pregnancy and after. These changes can help with behavior by consolidating brain growth, although their direct connection with ADHD is still being studied. We have many questions to answer:

- How much does a woman's diet during pregnancy affect the likelihood that her baby will end up having ADHD?

- What about the father's diet before conception?

- Is diet a direct cause of negative epigenetic changes that increase the risk of ADHD, or is it some other factor commonly associated with certain dietary habits?

- What dietary measures can pregnant women take to compensate for other harms that might contribute to ADHD (and other health risks for the baby)?

- Can a child's diet in early life compensate for prenatal dietary (or other) risks and protect a child from ADHD?

FAT INTAKE AND OBESITY DURING PREGNANCY

Some of the best evidence we have of a link between maternal diet and a child's ADHD comes from studies of fat intake and maternal metabolic state—in particular, increased inflammation—which are associated with the risk of obesity in offspring but also with offspring behavior, temperament, and neurodevelopmental disorders including ADHD. According to one survey, if a mother is obese, her child's chance of having ADHD triples. More studies will likely lower that startling estimate, but it seems clear we will end up with a confirmed association. Effects from maternal obesity in pregnancy or excess intake of "bad" fats (common in our society) during pregnancy contribute to what is called "metabolic syndrome" in children, placing them at risk for obesity and other ills—of which ADHD and irritable temperament may be one effect, at least in susceptible children.

It's important to understand, however, that a lot of scientific evidence that links diet to disease does not necessarily prove that elements of diet were a direct cause. All that might be observed is a correlation; for example, women under more stress or economic hardship may more easily gain excess weight as well as have offspring with attention problems. It may seem like the mother's obesity increased the risk of her child's ADHD, but it may have been that the stress she suffered was the key.

To unravel causality, a recent study in monkeys showed that if mothers ate a high-fat diet (that is, a diet just like the typical American's), their children had worse (irritable) temperaments as well as worse physical health. They also showed that the effect was related to epigenetic changes, first in the placenta and then in the child's brain, that affected neurotransmitters governing attention and mood, such as serotonin. (This was done by examining the animals' brains after they died.)

Unfortunately, we know little about the role of paternal diet or obesity, but I suspect, based on the existing literature on paternal effects from stress and chemical exposure, that it will prove to matter as well. Stay tuned to the research.

MICRONUTRIENTS AND BRAIN GROWTH

Omega-3s are not the only nutrient involved epigenetically in brain growth. It turns out that most of the positive effects on brain growth exerted by nutrients occur epigenetically, particularly in the prenatal period, and these nutrients include the micronutrients zinc, folate, vitamin B_{12}, vitamin A, and iron in addition to macronutrients like omega-3s. Variation in these nutrients affects not only a baby's brain growth but also temperament. For example, a series of studies by a nutrition research group in India, led by Sadhana Joshi, showed that maternal intake of folate and vitamin B_{12} led to epigenetic and thus developmental changes in several neurotransmitters in the offspring. It remains unclear how great all of these particular effects will prove to be on actual behavior

(ADHD), but it is clear that this direction needs to be explored and likely plays at least some role.

THE GOOD NEWS: FIGHTING "BAD" DIET WITH "GOOD"

Women expecting a child can feel tremendous pressure to protect their unborn child from harm and try to control what is sometimes out of their control. The good news, however, is that there are things pregnant women can do that may very well confer some protection against ADHD in children who, by their genetic and epigenetic legacy, are susceptible. The even better news is that most of these protective dietary factors are already recommended for everyone's overall health and also recommended by obstetricians for all pregnancies:

Upping Omega-3 Fatty Acids

A pilot study indicated that if the same mothers in the monkey study just mentioned were fed sufficient doses of omega-3 fatty acids, their offspring were protected. Because these experiments can randomly assign the animals to different conditions, they can rule out simple genetic effects on behavior as explaining the results. Studies of rodents as well as monkeys suggest that sufficient maternal intake of "good fats" like omega-3 in pregnancy could restore the necessary nutritional and epigenetic balance and prevent the epigenetic and health effects on offspring of the typical high-fat diet, or of maternal overweight before or during pregnancy. If this is confirmed, it will provide hope in otherwise difficult circumstances.

Reducing Saturated Fats and Trans Fats

Even better, naturally, is reduced intake of the "bad fats" as well. These are the fats that tend to contribute to obesity and other health problems. All of us should keep an eye on our consumption of them.

Taking Prenatal Vitamins

This is one of the first bits of advice an obstetrician typically gives expectant mothers: take prenatal vitamins. The folic acid contained in these vitamins is very important here. (Caution: Check with your doctor before consuming a lot of folic acid; recent data suggest it may be risky for a certain group of women.) Considering their positive effects on brain growth, those prenatal vitamins are like gold.

DIET IN YOUR CHILD'S EARLY LIFE

If you have been through a pregnancy after being very overweight or think you ate too much of a high-fat diet, it's not too late to try to counteract possible inflammatory effects. Most of the data on compensating for the negative epigenetic effects of prenatal diet pertain to obesity and weight gain, but since these prenatal experiences have been linked to changes in temperament and attention, we can take hope across the board. On that front, the evidence from animal studies is quite promising in suggesting that restoring the proper balance of the hormone leptin early in life interrupts these inflammatory effects on child development (leptin imbalance is involved in obesity). While there are many ways to restore this balance for a child at risk for so-called metabolic syndrome, caution is in order: medical treatment with supplemental leptin can be damaging to the health of a normal child. The better answer could be something most health organizations already recommend:

Breastfeeding

The safest and simplest way for young mothers to counteract negative influences during pregnancy is by breastfeeding. Standard recommendations suggest you should breastfeed for at least six months. However, the American Academy of Pediatrics recommends that you breastfeed for twelve months (introducing other foods after six months of age as a complement, but not a replacement, for breast milk). Some literature, including our own studies, do show a correlation of more breastfeeding (especially past six months) with reduced ADHD, but we don't know if that is a causal effect. The World Health Organization (WHO) studies show that breastfed babies show a more gradual, healthy weight gain than formula-fed babies, and the WHO encourages breastfeeding as late as twenty-four months of age.

Omega-3 Supplements

Also, the child's diet may be able to overcome negative epigenetic effects of prenatal diet, at least in part, by once again supplementing with omega-3. We know omega-3 can help with ADHD, but we don't know if the effect is particularly important for kids with a family history of less-than-ideal diet. Happily, breast milk delivers a lot of omega-3s to babies.

For more intriguing speculation on how diet may affect brain growth by creating positive epigenetic change, see the box on the facing page.

 TAKE-HOME POINTS

Food and the Development of the Brain during Pregnancy and Early Life

Brain development and function are related to nutrition. Mounting scientific evidence shows that nutrition, gut health, and food quality probably affect:

- Neurodevelopmental conditions like ADHD
- Cognitive abilities like attention
- Mood, emotions, and problems like anxiety

Practically all growth of the brain and the development of temperament rely on a mix of genetic and environmental effects, and the environmental component operates partly via epigenetics. We are still learning how much these mechanisms can influence ADHD, but we do now know that at least some of the process influences ADHD.

Epigenetic effects are like the radio volume dial. They are stable changes but not irreversible. The next time you turn the dial, the music volume changes too. A further experience can reverse some epigenetic processes. The question is what specific experiences are needed to reverse particular influences on ADHD.

While most positive nutri-ent effects, including epigenetic

In addition to compensating for earlier harms caused by a poor diet, we'll see in Chapter 6 that nutrients may compensate for damage caused by other factors (chemical pollutants), again by changing epigenetic signaling.

🔍 WHAT CAN WE LEARN FROM STUDIES OF THE EFFECTS OF DIET ON OTHER BRAIN PROBLEMS?

Evidence that diet can reverse epigenetic changes that lead to problems with brain development (like ADHD) or overcome the effects of an earlier epigenetic change is still emerging, but we have encouraging examples in two studies published in late 2015:

High-Protein, Low-Fat Diets Controlling Seizures. The first study examined seizures (an obvious brain problem) in adult rodents. When the rats were fed a ketogenic diet (high protein, low fat), their seizure problems were largely controlled. This worked better than seizure medication, and by dissecting the brains of these rodents, scientists could see the diet worked by altering DNA methylation—that is, epigenetically.

Low-Calorie Diets Speeding Recovery from Concussion. The second study looked at concussion, again using rodents but this time with young rats. The animals ate either a calorie-restriction diet, a high-fat diet, or a normal diet. Those on the calorie-restriction diet recovered better from the concussion, and again this was explained by epigenetic changes in key brain regions found in dissection. Crucially for clinical application, the epigenetic effects were also seen in blood tests.

If these diet-induced epigenetic changes can cure seizures in adult rodents and speed up recovery from a concussion in juvenile rodents, then in principle they can do the same for brain problems that are less dramatic than seizures or concussions. While this remains to be demonstrated, proof of the principle is there. Further, the effects of diet on ADHD, discussed in the next section of this chapter, indicate that this can work in practice: dietary changes can change epigenetic programming in children with ADHD and improve their brain function, health, executive functioning, attention, and self-regulation to a measurable extent.

effects, are the natural outcome of healthy eating, they also compensate for earlier harms. Whether during or after pregnancy, diet is worth looking at to maintain your child's neurodevelopmental (and overall) health and undo possible prior damage.

You have options for protecting your child through diet at each stage from pregnancy through early life and the rest of childhood. See the following action steps.

AT A GLANCE

Dietary Action Steps for Pregnancy and Early Life

If you are pregnant or planning to get pregnant:

- Do your best to keep your weight gain within the range recommended by your doctor.

- Increase your intake of omega-3 through diet or supplements (see specifics on page 64).

If you already have a child with ADHD:

- Consider breastfeeding (or feeding pumped breast milk) for the first twelve months, which may help counteract negative epigenetic effects of prenatal diet or obesity, although the benefit in preventing ADHD is still not well studied.

- Consider omega-3 supplementation. We don't yet know if it can ease the specific epigenetic effects of the mother's diet, but this is a fascinating possibility. Near future work should help clarify which children with ADHD particularly will benefit from omega-3 supplementation and whether this is related to prenatal diet exposures.

> A mother's diet may help protect the child from ADHD, and attention to the diet of a child who has ADHD might prove to reduce the effects of the disorder.

Diet and the Child with ADHD

As we've discussed, brain development begins before birth and continues throughout childhood and into young adulthood. It's never too late to "feed" your child's brain healthful nutrients. And we have some evidence that doing so can improve the symptoms of ADHD and poor self-regulation. So if your child has been diagnosed with ADHD or is showing some of the signs, it's prudent to look at his diet.

Let's start with common sense: If a child is overweight, eating empty calories, or not getting good nourishment, she will be more tired, listless, and unmotivated, won't feel good, and won't feel like focusing on schoolwork. You likely have seen this yourself in your own children or others. If your child is eating too much junk food—processed, filled with additives, and containing sugar (in all its myriad forms)—her energy is likely to be inconsistent and her mood less mellow. These effects alone can in turn make self-regulation challenging. And all of this is on top of diet's direct effects on ADHD and self-regulation specifically.

The suggestions you might encounter for dietary or nutritional help for ADHD are myriad. They run the gamut from well supported and advisable to poorly supported and even dangerous. Among the various proposals that parents have to navigate are:

- Single-nutrient supplements (for example, zinc, iron, magnesium, amino acids, vitamin D, calcium, carnitine, DMAE, or deanol)
- Omega-3 fatty acid (fish oil) supplements
- Multinutrient or super-nutrient supplementation
- Avoiding specific additives (for example, food coloring or sugar)
- Restriction or elimination diets ("few foods diet," "ketogenic diet," "Feingold diet")
- Probiotic supplementation

Obviously, any dietary changes you choose to make will depend on the cost–benefit ratio: how much help your child might get for the trouble it takes to make the change. I've arranged the possibilities starting with what's usually easiest (adding) and proceeding to what's a little harder (eliminating) and finally getting to the trickier options. How severe your child's problems are and how strong the scientific evidence is for the beneficial effect of a change will undoubtedly factor into your decisions. We again follow the principle that if it is safe, easy, and sensible, we require less evidence for accepting the idea than if it is risky, difficult, or expensive.

WHAT SHOULD I ADD?

Omega-3s

Omega-3s are found in most kinds of fish, eggs, olive oil, avocados, and other foods. When we were evolving, our diet probably included a lot more omega-3 fatty acid foods, so the ratio between different kinds of fat in our blood (such as omega-3, omega-6, and others) was a lot different than it is today. Over the last hundred years, at least in the West, the average diet has shifted toward a lot fewer of the foods that have omega-3s. Our own study, pooling data from over a dozen controlled studies, showed that children with ADHD tend to have low blood levels of omega-3s, although data from children in the United States remain sparse.

We also pooled results of over a dozen controlled trials in which children with ADHD and typically developing children were given omega-3 supplements. We found that there was a reliable benefit— although it was small. A major summary published in 2014 in *Child and Adolescent Psychiatric Clinics of North America* concluded that omega-3 supplementation is now an established intervention for children with ADHD. Other reviews have reached the same conclusions. These effects might be improved as more refined studies determine which combination of omega-3 and other fatty acids (such as omega-6), and which ratios of them, actually drive this initial effect.

> *Pooling data over more than a dozen controlled trials showed a composite 20 percent reduction in ADHD symptoms from omega-3 supplements.*

Although the effect was real, it is too small to be a total cure. This means that for most children the benefit will not be enough all by itself to "cure" ADHD or to be sufficient as a stand-alone treatment. It could still be of great value, however, because it might mean your child can get by with less medication. For some children, as well, benefits in terms of better mood and less irritability may be bigger than the effects on inattention alone, although the limited meta-analyses to date do not indicate better effects for other behaviors.

Risks and Side Effects. For children, the risks of omega-3 supplementation are that fish oil tablets can cause stomach upset, headache, insomnia, temporary diarrhea, or elevated blood readings of certain fats. One trial suggested about 5 percent of children experience one or more of these side effects. To prevent these effects, give the tablets with food and lower the dose if digestion problems occur. For pregnant women, the risks are subtler—check with your doctor before taking megadoses.

In fact, exactly what dose or type of omega-3 to give is not agreed on. The omega-3s include several compounds with acronyms like EPA and DHA. Our review suggested that EPA was the most important and that doses of 1,000 milligrams were more beneficial than lower doses, but that result was "soft" and could change with more research, and other reviews offer slightly different suggestions. The good news is that there is almost no risk to adding more of these fats to your child's diet other than stomach upset or diarrhea at very high doses.

How to Add Omega-3s. In addition to health foods like olive oil, avocado, and cold-water fish, you can get extra omega-3 with a *high-quality* supplement. Quality may be important—one suggestion is to look for "USP Verified" on the label, which indicates it is refined for purity and certified by U.S. Pharmacopeia. Another is to visit the local health food store and speak to the purchaser for the supplements. These individuals are often in the store checking stock and will be happy to recommend a brand they believe is the highest in quality, based on their knowledge of supply chains and product origins. The best alternative is to help your child learn to love tuna, salmon, sardines, mackerel, and even omega-3-enriched eggs. These foods can easily provide as much omega-3 as the best supplements and in the best form possible—food. Eating these three times a week may be sufficient to achieve your goal, according to a recent expert review chapter in Barkley's fourth edition of *Attention-Deficit/Hyperactivity Disorder* (see Resources).

Iron, Zinc, Magnesium, and Vitamin D: Only If Your Child Is Deficient

Iron and zinc are crucial to cell signaling and efficient nervous system functioning. Your child needs the right amount. Although animal studies show that insufficiency in these nutrients can lead to epigenetic effects on development, human studies have failed to show convincingly that blindly giving iron or zinc supplements to all children with ADHD helps. Further, too much iron or zinc is dangerous. If your child is having symptoms of ADHD, especially if he is not eating nutritious foods, it may make sense to get his blood levels checked. A surprising number of children have low iron levels, especially during periods of rapid growth. If blood levels indicate a deficiency, then it makes sense to supplement, but only in collaboration with your doctor. Otherwise, proceed with caution or avoid supplements, as overdosing can be dangerous.

Vitamin D is not as risky, but the story is much the same. Many children, particularly in northern latitudes, including the northern third of the United States, have low vitamin D. But even in sunny climates, children are often indoors and do not get enough sunlight. It can make sense to get your child's vitamin D blood levels checked and supplement if indicated by test results. If levels are appropriate, though, there is no evidence that more is better for ADHD.

Probiotics: Logical and Low Risk but Unproven for ADHD

Due to the explosion of knowledge about the gut microbiome, interest in probiotics has soared. The microbiome influences activity of brain chemicals like GABA and serotonin that are involved in mood, coping, stress, and possibly ADHD as well. A few studies in humans do suggest treatment with probiotics has improved mood and coping. The fact that they may improve mood may be valuable for some children with ADHD. Despite this logic, no proper trials of probiotic supplements for ADHD exist. We have to conclude that probiotic supplementation has a chance of helping mood and coping and may help digestion, but we have no evidence that would enable us to recommend it for ADHD. If you are considering probiotics for your child, consult with a nutritionist or your doctor about an appropriate brand and dosage. You can obtain probiotics in many foods, such as yogurts with live cultures, or from supplements. While they are low risk, they can cause stomachache and diarrhea. So, proceed if you want, but monitor carefully. View this as an "unproven" assist for ADHD.

Other Single-Nutrient Supplements

Most other single-nutrient supplements are unproven, insufficiently studied, or in a few instances dangerous when it comes to ADHD. Thus, unless a physician identifies a nutrient or metabolic deficiency, I do not see convincing evidence to support supplementing with zinc, vitamin D, iron, calcium, or other single supplements. The one exception may be carnitine; a recent expert review concluded it was sufficiently safe and promising that it could be worth a try, but only for inattentive, nonhyperactive children.

WHAT SHOULD I ELIMINATE?

A Wheelbarrow Full of Sugar for Every Child

In 2010, a famous chef named Jamie Oliver produced a classic TED Talk that has been viewed over six million times, entitled "Teach Every Child about Food." The talk focuses on poor food knowledge and obesity in our society. At one point, to clarify how much sugar the average child ingests, he dumps on the stage a wheelbarrow full of sugar cubes. There is no question that the sugar intake of our children is way out of control—from the corn syrup in so many canned and boxed foods, juices, and drinks to the sugar added to snacks. This is clearly a serious contributor to poor child health, increasing the risk of obesity, diabetes, and future heart disease. Efforts by consumer advocates to have the amount of "added sugar" in a food put on the food label are clearly sensible. Meanwhile, you are well advised to minimize your child's intake of any food or drink with added sugar (on the ingredients label this includes high-fructose corn syrup and many others; see the box on the next page) and to be aware that many supposedly healthy juices, soups, and cereals also contain unacceptable amounts of added sugar or fructose. This caution makes sense for general health, not just for ADHD.

That said, the real question for many parents is whether day-to-day sugar intake is making their child hyperactive. Is it? Surely many parents think so. Parents report that they think their child eats sugar, becomes hyperactive, then has a sugar crash. What is the science? In today's world, we have to distinguish *acute* sugar intake from *chronic* sugar intake.

ADHD and Acute Sugar Intake. Elegant experimental studies in the 1980s and 1990s convinced scientists that acute sugar intake was not a cause of hyperactivity. In these studies, experimenters randomly assigned some children to eat food with sugar while other children were randomly assigned to eat food with just artificial sweetener (aspartame) for up to three weeks. These studies failed to observe meaningful changes in daily hyperactivity. In one study, parents who *believed* their children had eaten

AVOIDING ADDED SUGAR

New FDA labeling requirements imposed in May 2016 and taking effect in 2018 will make it easier to avoid added sugar. They will require clear labeling of the amount of "added sugar" in a processed food. But because many foods naturally contain sugar, it will still be confusing to figure out what you are getting in any packaged food compared to what the food naturally had in it. An issue of the *Harvard Health Letter* published in 2014 gave this handy list of the names for sugar you might see on food package labels:

agave nectar   high-fructose corn syrup
brown sugar   honey
cane crystals   invert sugar
cane sugar   lactose
corn sweetener   malt sugar
corn syrup   malt syrup
crystalline fructose   maltose
dextrose   maple syrup
evaporated cane juice   molasses
fructose   raw sugar
fruit juice concentrates   sucrose
glucose

sugar food rated them as more hyperactive—even when the children had not been given sugary food but food with aspartame instead. A pooling of twenty-three such studies in 1995 showed that there was no reliable overall effect of sugar on child hyperactivity, even if there were some children hidden in the group who were having a sugar response. Thus, sugar, while unhealthy, is not linked to short-term hyperactivity.

ADHD and Chronic Sugar Intake. We have discovered just in the last few years that ADHD and obesity are linked. Children with ADHD are more likely to also become obese, although generally not until adolescence or adulthood. Why?

One possibility is that too many empty calories contribute to both obesity and attention problems. Another is that early-life toxins like pollution exposure (see Chapter 6) contribute to both problems. Still another is a shared neurobiology. For example, a key brain chemical in both food craving and ADHD is dopamine. Dopamine deficiency in the brain is related to ADHD and also related to drug addiction as well as to excess food craving. A fourth possibility, and perhaps the simplest, is that behaviors related to ADHD, like impulsive eating, increase the risk of obesity.

Keeping all this in mind, chronic sugar intake can cause permanent metabolic changes in brain chemicals that respond to food and reward. Some scientists have *speculated* that chronic sugar intake is helping to cause ADHD. They point to the link between ADHD and obesity, the parallel increase in sugar intake and clinical identification rates of ADHD, and the biological plausibility of chronic sugar intake changing the brain chemistry related to reward (dopamine, just mentioned) in a way that is similar to what we see in ADHD. While this is a very interesting idea, it relies on what lawyers call a circumstantial argument. At the same time, it's what scientists call an interesting hypothesis.

 TAKE-HOME POINT

While we can't pin ADHD on sugar, given the risk–benefit ratio for overall health, getting a handle on your child's total added sugar intake is a good idea. The single best way to do this is to sharply limit soda, juice, and other artificial drinks, where many individuals get most of their added sugar. It is worth your while to look at labels and try to cut added sugar elsewhere as well as much as you can manage.

Avoid Caffeinated and Energy Drinks

Sugar isn't the only additive in drinks that parents now have to think about. Caffeine is popular in energy drinks and bars that children consume. Today's children typically are getting caffeine daily—even if parents are not tracking it. One recent national survey in the United States reported that nearly 75 percent of children and teens ingest some caffeine on a daily basis. This comes from sodas (like Mountain Dew and Coke), energy drinks, and, for teens, tea and coffee, as well as chocolates and sweets. How much caffeine your child gets can be deceptive. The box on the next page shows that two or three of the wrong sodas or one energy drink equals a 12-ounce cup of coffee! That's simply too much caffeine for a young child.

The American Academy of Pediatrics recommends that developing children completely avoid caffeine. (Canadian guidelines suggest a limit of 45 milligrams of caffeine a day—equal to one 12-ounce bottle of caffeinated soda or 4–6 ounces of regular coffee.) The health risks of too much caffeine are substantial for young children. These risks increase if children are taking ADHD medication, due to the unpredictability of the combined effects on heart rate and blood pressure. Even more serious is a remote but still increased chance of seizures in susceptible individuals. The side effects of too much caffeine are familiar to those of you who drink too much coffee—jitteriness, stomachache, headache, sleep problems, increased blood pressure. These effects can occur at very low doses in young children. For preadolescent children, it is prudent to prevent use of caffeinated beverages for health reasons.

HOW MUCH CAFFEINE IS MY CHILD GETTING?

Average amount of caffeine in common products[*]:

12 oz. drip coffee	140 mg
12 oz. decaffeinated coffee	3 mg
12 oz. tea	96 mg
12 oz. soda	40–100 mg
12 oz. Red Bull energy drink	140 mg

Recommended maximum daily intake:

Adults, "alertness dose" (per day)	50–300 mg
Adults, "recommended maximum" (Canada)	360 mg
Children, maximum (Canada)	45 mg
Children, maximum (U.S.)	0 mg

Actual daily intake average in the U.S.[*]:

Adults	300 mg
Children and teens	100 mg

[*]Source: U.S. Food and Drug Administration

Does Caffeine Contribute to ADHD? The updated scientific findings:

- Individuals with ADHD tend to consume more caffeine than non-ADHD individuals.

- Teens with ADHD are *twice* as likely as their peers to consume caffeine.

- The same is true of individuals with depression, substance use, and other problems.

- Caffeine in low to moderate doses can improve focus and alertness.

- Caffeine in high doses can lead to over-arousal and hyperactivity.

- Caffeine's individual effects depend on your genetic makeup. One important gene is the adenosine-2A gene.

Caffeine overdose is a risk for young people who consume too many energy drinks (one can be "one too many"), resulting in jitteriness and hyperactivity as well as inattention due to hyperarousal.

Can Caffeine Treat ADHD? The excess use of caffeine by individuals with ADHD may be a case of self-medicating. I have met individuals with ADHD, and even some parents, who think they can help ADHD by drinking coffee.

Here's how that might work. Part of caffeine's effect on alertness seems to be due to secondary release of dopamine in the brain—an effect that overlaps with the effect of stimulant medications, which also release dopamine in the brain, although via a different chemical route. In the 1970s and 1980s a small number of studies investigated whether caffeine (either in tablet form or as coffee) in doses of 150–200 milligrams per day could in fact alleviate symptoms of ADHD. An analysis of this literature at the end of the 1990s concluded that caffeine in this dose range probably had some beneficial effects on ADHD symptoms at least in the short run (that is, ignoring the rapid tolerance that can build up) but was not as effective as stimulant medication. Both subsequent and very recent studies in animals found some benefits of caffeine in learning and cognition. In the middle of the 2010s, this has led to renewed calls by some experts to reexamine the potential benefits of caffeine.

Given its benefits in terms of alertness and cognition, can it help children with ADHD? Perhaps, but don't bank on it. At this point, the research in this area is too limited for us to allow any conclusions from it. I don't advise caffeine as a treatment for your child, due to the risks, lack of reliable dosing guidelines, and lack of guidelines on frequency of administration or side effects of regular use at any dosages in children.

Artificial Food Additives

These are worth minimizing, but doing so is complicated, so I take this up again in the next section in the context of dietary changes generally.

MORE COMPLICATED ADDITIONS, SUBTRACTIONS, AND SUBSTITUTIONS

Organic Food

While the jury is still out as to how significant the role of pesticides is in children's brain development (see Chapter 6), if you want to be on the safe side, avoid foods with pesticide chemicals on or in them. You can do this simply by switching to all-organic produce, meat, and dairy. The catch: organic foods are typically more expensive. But even by mixing some organic foods into your diet you will reduce your child's body levels of pesticides. Studies have shown that within a few weeks of switching to an all-organic diet, the pesticide metabolites in children's urine drop dramatically. This isn't extra work—but it might take extra money. Still, the investment may be worth it compared to other ways to help your child.

Multinutrient or "Super-Nutrient" Supplementation

One promising new direction concerns *multinutrient supplements*—a pill with massive enriched supplementation of many vitamins and minerals. Such a supplement may achieve many of the benefits of a carefully controlled fresh food diet but be easier to handle. This approach makes sense in that nutrients naturally work in tandem, so supplementing with just one nutrient is unlikely to do very much. Preliminary studies in ADHD have been promising, and more are now under way. Future studies using this approach will be of keen interest, but this literature is still too small to confirm effects. Consider this "promising and possibly effective" but not established.

Restriction Diets and Food Additives

The most ambitious level of dietary intervention is also the one that has been recommended the longest and the one that has been the most controversial: a restriction diet to eliminate food allergens and synthetic food additives. These diets vary, and each study uses a somewhat different actual restriction diet. Overall, however, on such diets, some well-controlled studies report that ADHD symptoms are reduced from 10 to 100 percent. Others report that while ADHD symptoms don't improve much, mood and irritability do improve. Nearly every one of the few studies that have been done identifies at least a small group of parents who report their child is dramatically improved. Studies that "challenge" children with placebo-controlled trials of food additives show similar results—while effects range from nil to modest, studies consistently find a subgroup of "responders." In recent years (from 2012 to 2016) several meta-analyses of this small but important literature have updated our understanding. In this section we'll work through this complicated topic.

Some Definitions First. A restriction or elimination diet can come in numerous forms. The most intensive eliminates a wide range of potentially allergenic foods as well as food additives and then slowly adds them back in one by one to create a diet that does not provoke a reaction. These allergens and additives are clearly not specific to ADHD—but ADHD could be one of the many negative reactions that can occur in sensitive children.

It's helpful to trace the somewhat confusing history of controversy about food and ADHD. Related ideas about children's behavior problems date all the way to the 1920s, espoused at that time by a clinician named Albert Rowe among others. The idea was popularized in relation to ADHD in the 1970s by Benjamin Feingold, an allergist in Oakland. This diet is still promoted by the foundation he created and is easily

---

COMMON FOOD ADDITIVES

The degree of evidence linking additives to health or behavioral reactions is variable.

- Artificial colors
- Artificial flavors and flavor enhancers (monosodium glutamate [MSG] or monopotassium glutamate)
- Artificial sweeteners (aspartame, acesulfame K, neotame, saccharin, sucralose)
- Preservatives and stabilizers (sodium benzoate, butylated hydroxyanisole [BHA], butylated hydroxytoluene [BHT], carrageenan)
- Protein extenders (for example, hydrolyzed, textured, or modified protein)

---

found on the Internet. The idea was that food additives, particularly synthetic dyes and colorings, were triggering physical reactions in children and causing hyperactivity. He recommended a restriction diet in which all allergenic foods and food dyes were to be removed from the child's diet. Let's pause and break this down.

According to allergists, reactions to food or food ingredients take two forms.

- A *food allergy* is an immunological reaction after eating a food. It can cause headache, runny nose, GI upset or other problems, skin irritation, and other symptoms. These reactions occur soon after eating the offending food—that is, typically within the same day.

- *Food sensitivity* is a nonimmunological response to a food item. It is theorized to be due to enzyme deficiency (as in lactose intolerance) or another direct toxic reaction. Food sensitivities are difficult to pin down because the response is subtler and can occur days or even weeks after eating the food. In the case of ADHD, at least, specific biological mechanisms of food intolerance are difficult to demonstrate.

Although Feingold proposed that ADHD resulted from a food allergy, other proponents suggest that ADHD is related to food or additive sensitivity. A food allergy is easier to spot than a food sensitivity because a food allergy usually causes some sort of response shortly after the food was eaten, and a food sensitivity may take days or weeks to manifest.

A restriction or elimination diet attempts to address a food allergy or sensitivity by eliminating offending foods and then replacing them one by one to diagnose and treat the problem. It can range from eliminating a single food (as in a wheat-free diet) to several specific foods, as in the six-food elimination diet (eliminating common allergenic foods—soy, wheat, eggs, seafood, cow milk protein, and peanuts), to the "few foods" (oligoantigenic) diet, which allows only a few restricted foods deemed to have low allergenic potential.

Several studies, in the 1970s and 1980s, small by today's standards, investigated the possible effects of synthetic food dyes as well as the benefits of a restriction diet based on Feingold's recommendations or a few-foods diet. Some were laborious—taking all the food out of the house and making sure children and families ate only the food prepared by the researchers. Others used disguised juice or cookies to test children's reactions with and without eating food dyes or other "food challenge" ingredients. They then looked at parent ratings, teacher ratings, and in some cases children's performance on tests of attention in the laboratory. Some studies looked at same-day reactions for an allergenic response. Others looked at response over several weeks to evaluate food sensitivities.

The results were decidedly mixed. In 1983 the first major review concluded that the effects of food dyes on behavior were trivial and the

---

FAQ: WHICH FOODS ARE ALLERGENIC?

The six common allergenic foods eliminated in a six-food elimination diet:

- Eggs
- Wheat
- Soy
- Cow milk protein
- Peanuts
- Seafood

Some lists add tree nuts (walnuts, cashews) and separate shellfish from other seafood.

benefits of a restriction diet were minimal. For many years this was the consensus among scientists. However, in the late 1990s and early 2000s, additional studies and reviews emerged, including the first large, randomized population study, done in England. (In the Introduction I defined the different types of research studies, but the box on the facing page goes into more detail on why the randomized double-blind controlled study is the gold standard.)

These began to show a more nuanced picture. My colleagues and I conducted our own careful reanalysis of this literature using newer meta-analytic statistical methods in 2012, pooling results of all double-blind, randomized studies over the past thirty-five years. Our results were like those of other reviews conducted at that time and subsequently. The following are the key conclusions reached by us and by others.

- Artificial food dyes and/or preservatives cause a small increase in ADHD symptoms, including a short-term (presumably allergenic) response in a minority of children with ADHD and in some non-ADHD children.

- A restriction and elimination diet or a few-foods diet carried out over several weeks causes a small overall improvement in ADHD symptoms, and a large improvement in a small minority of children.

- Although food dyes and/or preservatives have a worsening effect on ADHD symptoms overall, the diet restriction benefit is not due mostly to food dyes. It is due also to other additives and thus most likely to a range of food allergies and sensitivities in the population, which may vary from child to child.

- We do not have a good method for identifying in advance which children will respond by showing fewer ADHD symptoms or mood symptoms.

- Food sensitivity is more likely than food allergy as a contributor to ADHD.

- Conclusions are "soft"—only a small number of well-controlled trials have been conducted. One or two large studies could weaken some conclusions.

FAQ: HOW DO I KNOW A STUDY ON THE CAUSE
OF ADHD IS RELIABLE?

The following are the major considerations for a scientific design.

1. Are the measures valid—for example, was ADHD carefully defined? Was diet carefully measured? A clinic study may have far better measurement than a national survey.

2. How generalizable is the sample? For example, a study of children referred to a clinic may be biased because only children with insurance and multiple problems come in for care. A national survey may have far better generalizability than a clinic study.

3. Is the study causal or correlational? As I've explained, correlation is not causation. Different studies give different levels of confidence.

   a. A cross-sectional, correlational study observes that children who have ADHD also have some other characteristic, like low blood levels of vitamin D. But this does not prove that one caused the other. Kids with ADHD might stay indoors more and thus have less vitamin D, or a third factor not measured, such as living in a region with a dark climate and limited health care, might explain both points.

   b. A prospective study controls for what came first. Children are enrolled before they have ADHD or an exposure, and the outcomes are looked at. For example, children might be enrolled at birth and their existing lead level measured. Then subsequent lead exposure is measured, and after that, ADHD outcome. These are stronger than simple cross-sectional studies.

   c. "Natural experiments" provide even more hints about causation. For example, researchers can see whether ADHD is more likely to occur after smoking by surrogate mothers who are not genetically related to the child.

   d. The gold standard for causality is called a double-blind, randomized controlled trial. It has the following elements:

   • There are at least two conditions (such as treatment, no treatment).

   • Participants are assigned to a condition by a random process (a coin toss or a random number generator).

   • The participants do not know what condition they are assigned to—the conditions are disguised (single blind). This requires a

carefully designed placebo or no-treatment condition. For example, in a diet study, children get two identical-looking and -tasting
foods with different ingredients.

- The experimenter does not know what condition each person is
  assigned to (double blind). This is done by having a third party
  randomize and assign people to conditions.

- The experimenter faithfully carries out the comparison that was
  planned before the study began and does not invent new comparisons after the fact (which can create chance findings).

- When all of these steps are successfully followed, and the double
  blind is verified successful, there is no other explanation for a finding than that it was caused by the treatment condition. Unmeasured factors are randomized out, so they can't explain the effect.

Food Dyes and Allergies: The Practical Upshot? You can avoid or
reduce food additives by focusing on nonprocessed foods (fresh produce,
fresh meat, and whole-grain breads and pastas). Here are some rules of
thumb suggested by nutritionist colleagues:

- Read labels, and if you see ingredients that you're not familiar
  with, don't have in your kitchen, or would not use in your own
  cooking, don't buy the food.

- To find fresh food, shop the outside aisles of the supermarket.

- To avoid allergenic foods, replace foods with nonallergenic sub-
  stitutes.

- Consult a nutritionist before embarking on a full restriction/elimi-
  nation diet (otherwise, you risk malnourishing your child).

- Before making a major dietary change, be sure your child will
  comply with it—you may need to address parent–child issues first
  (see Chapter 8).

Our analysis, while on a limited body of work, still suggested as a
best guess about a 30 percent chance that your child will respond posi-
tively to a major dietary effort in terms of tolerating the diet and seeing
at least some gains in attention and behavior.

The Catch: This Ain't Easy. The catch to this approach is it is hard to do—many children don't like the alternatives. So you have to make changes gradually, and you may have to find a way to motivate your child with a reward plan or behavior plan (see Chapter 8). Also, if you eliminate lots of foods, you **must** consult with a nutritionist, or you will risk causing nutritional deficiencies in your child.

 TAKE-HOME POINTS

Diet and the Child with ADHD

Most of the food suggestions in this chapter are sensible for all kids. But if your child has ADHD, you have less margin for error. For many kids, a typical modern diet with all its shortcomings may be relatively harmless—they have lucky genetics, their body compensates, and they get by. But for kids with ADHD, the body may be very much like the mind—very reactive to the environment. If your child has ADHD, it makes

> *For children with ADHD, the body may be very reactive to the environment, just as their mind is.*

sense to get every advantage you can. It now looks like paying attention to diet is worth it, at least in part.

So if you think food is playing a role in your child's problems, you may be right! Recent work has overturned prior skepticism about the value of nutrition or diet in ADHD. We now know that omega-3 supplementation benefits children with ADHD—although in most cases it's not a big enough effect to replace other treatments.

 AT A GLANCE

Food and ADHD Action Steps

The Fundamentals

You've heard all this before, but now your understanding of the gut–brain axis may underscore the importance of focusing on nutrients (macro and micro):

1. Minimize fast food: cook at home (and keep it simple to avoid driving yourself crazy) or get good-quality prepared meals elsewhere most days.
2. Provide plenty of fresh fruits and vegetables.
3. Minimize processed food.
   a. Use whole grains instead of processed or refined grains.
   b. Minimize junk food, soda, or juices that include any type of sugar in the label.

The Specifics

Stay fresh. Shift your family to more fresh fruits and vegetables; minimize boxed and packaged food products.

Shop outside. Shop the outside aisles of the store to avoid processed food.

Go organic. To avoid pesticide residue, supplements, and additives, buy organic foods.

Sardines are your friend. Eat plenty of cold-water fish to get omega-3 fatty acids or choose a high-quality purified (USP-labeled) fish oil supplement with 1–2 grams of omega 3, at least half EPA. (Unfortunately, scientific-sounding claims for various omega-3-type products are rife on the Internet; ask your health-food store buyer to suggest a high-quality product.)

Monitor allergens. Avoid allergenic foods if your child shows any reactions.

Check blood levels. Ask your doctor to check your child's blood levels of iron, zinc, vitamin D, or other minerals as well as omega-3s during routine physicals.

Sugar. Although not specific to ADHD, sugar is a major health risk. Sharply limit added sugar and sugary drinks.

Caffeine. Eliminate caffeine for preadolescent or growing children.

Probiotics. These are unproven for ADHD but healthy overall: check with your doctor and start slow.

Don't sweat the rest. Ignore the maze of other dietary suggestions for ADHD.

The good news here is that the upshot—to get your family on a healthy diet—is a good idea even if you aren't sure it will help with ADHD. We don't need ADHD research to carry out the suggestions here—they all make good health sense for everyone. What's new is the recognition that ADHD itself can improve.

> *The dietary principles we now know can help improve (or prevent) ADHD are good for the overall health of your child and your entire family.*

Simply by moving your family to a healthy diet of fresh foods prepared (as much as possible) and eaten at home, cutting out sugary drinks and processed food, and eating organic fruits and vegetables (to avoid pesticide residues and because they are usually fresher), you can achieve a great deal. That approach will increase

---

HOW DO YOU GET CHILDREN TO EAT HEALTHY FOODS?

One of the most pernicious myths is that children who will not eat healthy food have to be given "something" that they will eat. Science does not bear this out. What experiments show is that if all the choices given to children are healthy, children will choose one of the options and eat it. Example: Snacks may be carrots, apple slices, nuts, or cheese. Drink choices can be water or milk (no sugary drink). A child may complain the first day the "new options" come into effect, but ultimately the child will eat—he will not starve himself. You can just matter-of-factly provide the available options. You can't rely on children's "instinct" for choosing healthy food or getting the nutrients they need when unhealthy food is available. Their bodies are smart but evolved before processed food. Their instincts don't know how to filter healthy from unhealthy food if it is tasty. Even mice become malnourished when offered sugary along with healthy food. The keys:

- Provide choices.
- Provide only healthy choices.
- If all the choices are healthy, then kids can pretty much eat what they want.

nutrient value, avoid additives like food coloring that can contribute to ADHD, and reduce total sugar intake for your child. If you include plenty of cold-water fish, your child will get ample omega-3 fatty acids as well. The principal additions that are ADHD specific are to make sure to get the omega-3 fatty acids and have your doctor check your child's blood levels of iron, zinc, and vitamin D if there is any doubt about those nutrients.

4

Exercise, Sleep, and ADHD
New Insights on Brain Growth

Science has now absorbed the reality that the brain is malleable and "plastic." That means the brain can to a surprising extent "reinvent itself" with learning, experience, or the right stimulation. We also now know that epigenetic changes in the brain help it do that. The limits on this ability and its sensitivity remain open frontiers for investigation. As a result, we're experiencing an explosion of scientific interest in whether we can build up attention and executive function, even self-regulation and behavioral control, by stimulating changes in gene expression in the brain. How far can we go with changes in lifestyle that also might stimulate epigenetic change? It turns out that, besides nutrition and diet, two major lifestyle activities that also affect general health are particularly relevant to growing exactly the parts of the brain that strengthen self-regulation, and thus can help counteract or improve ADHD. They are **exercise** and **sleep**. Getting exercise and getting enough sleep are obviously good for general health and good for all children. But for kids with ADHD, they may have specific benefits that are well worth your time.

Exercise

The benefits of exercise and overall fitness are well established for general health, mood, and stress management. These perks are increasingly popularized in the media. For example, *Time's* cover story in September

2016 was on exercise as a medicine—highlighting the view of some specialists that exercise can be more effective than most drugs for many health conditions. But what is the real benefit for children, in particular for those with ADHD? How important is this particular lifestyle option? With the advent of studies that combine exercise and brain imaging, we are learning exactly what exercise can do for brain growth. And recent clinical trials have just started to determine to what extent exercise can help children with ADHD. While these are early days, the future is likely to bring further positive evidence.

Particularly interesting for ADHD in recent years is a series of findings showing that for developing children aerobic exercise expands the growth of brain connections, the frontal cortex, and the brain chemicals (such as serotonin and dopamine) that support self-regulation and executive functioning. These surprisingly specific findings in typically developing children have led to real excitement about the possibility that the right kind of exercise can help ADHD. We'll dig into this evidence, evaluate it, and sort out what kind of exercise is best based on the findings of just the last five years.

EXERCISE VERSUS SPORTS VERSUS "FREE PLAY"

But first a couple of preliminary considerations. We need to sort out exercise from its overlap with "free play" and "sports." Free play is essential; exercise is beneficial; sports are optional. Free play has its own inherent benefits independent of any exercise. Recent findings confirm that it helps children develop problem solving, coping skills, imagination, and self-directed learning. For preschool children, most free play involves large-motor activity and so is ideal for their development. However, for school-age children, free play is often less active. It remains just as important for other reasons. We don't know, however, if free play has any special importance for children with ADHD.

Sports, likewise, have a different set of benefits. They may provide exercise, although this varies with the sport. They can also promote self-discipline and provide camaraderie and social experience, and for children with ADHD who are good at the sport, a source of protective self-esteem. For some children with ADHD, athleticism is a compensating strength and an arena where they can gain some positive self-image to offset their struggles in school. For others with ADHD who are not so gifted or inclined, sports can be an extremely frustrating and unhappy experience.

Vigorous exercise is critical to the developing brain—especially when ADHD is hindering that development—but don't assume that team sports are the only (or the best) choice for your child.

Either way, sports that involve a lot of waiting may not do enough for the brain or for fitness. Some sports are great for fitness: one-on-one racquetball, basketball, soccer, high-activity dancing, bicycling, running—in these sports there's plenty of vigorous exercise. In contrast, just playing nine-on-nine baseball, golfing with a cart, or eleven-on-eleven American football might not bring enough fitness, unless accompanied by a practice regimen that enforces fitness.

Keep in mind that children's fitness habits can stay with them into adulthood. If you played soccer throughout your childhood and adolescence, you might very well seek out an adult soccer league to play in. But for most adults, team sports are logistically challenging. That's why most adults in our society stay fit through individual exercise. Exercise is a good habit to instill early in life, not just because cardio and strength/flexibility training will be key to adult health, but because in childhood *cognitive and motor development work in tandem.* In the brain, extensive connections wire motor centers, like the cerebellum and the motor cortex, to areas involved in attention and executive functioning, like the prefrontal cortex and the basal ganglia. Some physiologists believe that for the best cognitive and self-regulation outcomes for kids, exercise should include complex motor learning and coordination—that is, general motor skill growth along with aerobic challenge. For preschoolers, this may naturally occur in their running, climbing, and wrestling around during free play. But for older children, it may require an organized activity, either individually or with a partner or a team. These might include activities like rock climbing, dance, basketball, or martial arts. Here again, you'll have to use some judgment to balance free play and structured activity. If your teenager is choosing her own activity for Saturday afternoon and decides to go rock climbing with a qualified supervisor, her free play and ideal exercise may be one and the same. On the other hand, if your ten-year-old chooses to use his free play time to build a model with Legos, or to read, draw, or play with low-key games with friends outside, then he may need in addition to go for a vigorous bike ride or play a sport.

Before we focus on ADHD-related exercise benefits, therefore, put them in the context of these guidelines:

 AT A GLANCE

Action Steps for Choosing the Best Exercise

1. Group sports should be considered *optional,* and decisions made about enrolling your child in a specific sports program should be based on:

   • The level of vigorous exercise (breathing harder, heart rate up)

   • Your child's ability to enjoy the sport. If your child is thriving in a particular sport, encourage it. If he hates it, let him do something else.

2. Always allow your child with ADHD enough free play (active or not), adding exercise on top of free play if necessary.

3. The main thing is to get the exercise, which can be done in a lot of different ways. Stay open.

EXERCISE, EPIGENETICS, AND THE BRAIN

Exercise is one of the lifestyle factors with the clearest epigenetic effects. A sustained fitness program, at any age, causes *significant epigenetic changes* throughout the *body* (some of which are obvious, like heart and muscle genes) but, it turns out, also *in the brain.* The brain growth effects, under study for the past several years, now have a sufficiently large literature to be considered definite. They were confirmed in comprehensive scientific reviews in 2013 and 2014.

The *epigenetic* effects on the brain are still being studied, but evidence so far is quite positive here as well. Animal studies suggest that exercise triggers epigenetic changes such as histone modifications or DNA methylation that specifically alter activity in genes that influence new neuron growth and extend neural dendritic connections. In plain English, this means that *exercise can exert effects that make the brain grow more and get more efficient.* Even more encouraging regarding ADHD is that this seems to happen in particular brain areas like the hippocampus, basal ganglia, and frontal cortex, which are fundamental to self-regulation and executive functioning. In these animal studies mice either exercise vigorously or not, and then are examined for brain growth, gene expression, and epigenetic changes. Do such animal studies prove that children who exercise will get the same benefits? It's a bit of a stretch, but actually it doesn't get much better than this as far as effects we would want to see in an animal model go. So these studies, while preliminary, are

> *Exercise positively affects precisely the areas of the brain that control the functions at the heart of ADHD: self-regulation and executive skills.*

extremely encouraging. Let's look at the effects of exercise on children in three areas most relevant to ADHD: learning, attention, and ADHD symptoms.

Exercise and Academics/Learning

One of the biggest reasons that inattention is a problem is it interferes with academics. In fact, my colleagues and I, and many others, have shown that attentional control, self-regulation, and executive function are the most important predictors of academic success—more important than IQ or behavioral problems. For kids with ADHD, academic problems are the number one complaint along with behavioral problems. Therefore, one of the most important areas for us to look at with exercise is whether it helps kids with their academics, and in particular with the executive function part of academic success.

Fortunately, developmental studies of child exercise have used academic results as a primary focus (in part because school PE programs make it a natural place to do safe, controlled experiments). Despite this, the caveat is that this literature is still short on very-high-quality randomized trials of the sort that provide the acid test of exercise benefits. However, a major monograph published in 2014 by the Society for Research in Child Development concluded that overall, exercise led to improved academic performance in children—*more than equivalent additional class or study time.* In other words, school poli-

> *Cutting phys ed classes in favor of academics is enormously self-defeating for child learning.*

cies to cut physical education classes are a mistake. The science indicates that schools should convert physical education classes into physical fitness classes and keep them going.

Exercise and Attention/Executive Functions

Testifying to the explosion of interest in this area, the years 2013, 2014, 2015, and 2016 each saw updated scientific reviews in which experts assembled all available studies to see if exercise actually improved the mental abilities necessary for self-regulation that are typically impaired in ADHD. One in the *Annual Review of Psychology* (2014) concluded that typically developing children show better attention and executive function on the day they exercise—suggesting exercise prior to going to school could be useful. Altogether these authoritative reviews lead to the following conclusions:

- Fitness is associated with better child working memory, response inhibition, and learning.
- This holds up clearly in large correlational studies but is also supported in the more informative prospective and randomized controlled studies.

We definitely need more randomized trials to gain confidence here, but if we try to peer into the future, the most likely picture is that exercise improves attention and even executive functioning in typically developing children and therefore directly counteracts ADHD by building self-regulation in the brain. Until the 2010s, we had no direct data, however, on whether ADHD itself would improve with exercise. Now such data is finally emerging, albeit slowly.

Exercise and ADHD

Over two dozen studies now have evaluated whether children with ADHD benefit from an exercise program. Unfortunately, these studies are all very small and riddled with inconsistency and methodological limitations, so this is not yet a "mature" literature that allows confident conclusions. But they let us begin, in Gretzky's words, to "skate to where the puck is going," and see what the most likely future picture will be. Between 2014 and 2016, three scientific reviews attempted to quantify the actual benefits of exercise programs across all studies as a treatment for ADHD, and a fourth summarized a larger number of studies that could not be pooled due to their differences in approach. A 2015 meta-analysis (statistical summary of all studies) found seven small studies of aerobic fitness in ADHD. These were all flawed in some way (for example, none were able to clearly disguise from the participants what condition they were in, leading to possible expectation effects or compliance effects) and small (fewer than fifty kids, increasing the risk of a chance finding or of finding exaggerated effects). In other words, they may overestimate effects. In particular, lack of clear blinding of observers is a problem because it means that observers' own beliefs and expectations will influence the results. All were short term (three studies ran for one week, three ran for five to six weeks, and one ran for ten weeks)—effects might take longer to take hold. However, with these cautions in mind, the pooled data were still encouraging: benefits on hyperactivity, attention, executive function, and cognition equaled about half the effect of medication—and were greater than the effect of diet—for the children with ADHD. In other words, these effects were big enough that you would notice them in everyday life. Based on the history of diet research,

> Current research, while still preliminary, does suggest that aerobic exercise can provide noticeable improvements in ADHD symptoms—about half as much as medication but possibly more than dietary changes. Larger studies in the future will likely confirm the effects but show that they're not quite as strong as we've seen so far.

what's likely is that subsequent larger studies will confirm these effects are real, while ultimately finding that the size of the effect is a bit less than claimed in the 2015 paper. The much larger review of studies in 2016, while it did not pool the results, drew the conclusion that aerobic exercise yielded a believable benefit for children with ADHD—both in their symptoms and in their overall health. Strength-building exercise (such as yoga, tai chi, weights, CrossFit, or others) is not sufficiently well studied yet to draw conclusions about it.

Caveats: What We Still Don't Know

Which kinds of exercises don't help the brain? Most research has been on cardio (aerobic) exercise. What about strength training or other types of exercise? Work on this is just beginning. How permanent are benefits in children? Most studies are on adults, and most experimental trials with children have been pretty limited. What is the benefit of sustained fitness programs (as opposed to same-day or same-week benefit) for kids with ADHD? This has not yet been studied. How big are individual differences? Should different kids with different genetic makeups have different kinds of exercise to maximize their brain growth and attention? This new area is important. Like everything else in this book, it won't end up being one size fits all. A particular question is whether boys and girls benefit from the same activities; most studies to date have been on boys.

As with muscles, the effects of exercise on the brain depend on keeping at it over time.

How long should you continue the fitness program to help treat ADHD? It's unknown. Even a week can help—but only temporarily. Even though exercise causes epigenetic changes, it takes sustained exercise over time for those to build up to a noticeable influence on growth. Truly growing the brain is like growing the muscles—it requires sustained fitness, suggesting you should maintain the effort over several weeks or months.

TAKE-HOME POINTS

Exercise and ADHD

If your child has ADHD, the benefits of exercise are even more important than for other kids. The unique effects of exercise on the brain networks and gene expression patterns that support maturation of self-regulation should make you sit up and take notice.

- Exercise and fitness have a nice side effect of protecting your child from serious health problems (like obesity and diabetes), improving health in such areas as skin, muscle, and bone, and improving coordination, while advancing your goal of brain growth in systems that support self-regulation and help combat ADHD.

- With epigenetic effects involved, developmental effects may well be sustained even during years that exercise slacks off—we are still learning how many effects are short term versus long term in this regard.

- A final benefit shown in studies is that exercise is a powerful route to creating epigenetic change that can overcome negative events earlier in life. For example, animal studies have reported that exercise can prevent or reverse the epigenetic effects of stress and trauma in early life—the topic of our next chapter.

- A good diet provides more energy for exercise as well.

- Exercise can be fun—it's sometimes a matter of finding the right outlet to pique your child's interests. For some families, it helps to exercise with your child—a shared bike ride, hike, run, or game.

✓   **AT A GLANCE**

Exercise and ADHD Action Steps

On several occasions in the past decade, scientists have surveyed the landscape for typically developing children. Lacking ADHD-specific guidelines, our best bet is to go with these general guidelines but to highlight their likely extra relevance to children with ADHD, who need every boost they can get in relation to learning, attention, executive function, and self-regulation. Here are the general and most common recommendations.

Make sure your child gets at least one hour a day of moderate and moderate-to-intensive exercise (heart rate up and breathing a bit harder). It doesn't have to be all at once. It can be one sixty-minute period, two thirty-minute periods, or four fifteen-minute periods. (These guidelines come from the American Heart Association.) Some children need more exercise than others. Some children may be happier and calmer if they can get two hours a day, but even some exercise will help their health and mood.

If realistically feasible, try for the main exercise at the beginning of the day so your child is ready for the school day. While difficult to arrange, some schools and some families have been able to do this. It's the ideal! However, obviously that won't be possible for everyone. Most kids will have to go to school and then get their exercise after school, in addition to what we all hope is recess time.

Make sure the exercise includes a mix of moderate activity (walking, level bicycling, roller blading, skateboarding, jumping rope, playing on the playground) and moderate to intense activity sufficient to make the child huff and puff or break a sweat (running, cycling on hills, swimming, vigorous dancing, martial arts, soccer, basketball, playing chase, gymnastics, sustained calisthenics). (These recommendations come from the British National Health Service.) The activity should be consistent during the time period—don't count activities that include a lot of standing around or waiting for a turn.

Include activities that involve motor skill learning and coordination—that is, some cognitive challenge. While the extra benefits of this approach are not yet definitive, it is possible that added brain growth happens here. Most ball sports involve at least some motor learning, while dance, martial arts, rock climbing, gymnastics, CrossFit, or some calisthenics like jump rope may entail more complete whole-body muscle learning.

It's okay to mix activities; you don't have to hit all aspects every day. For example, your child may like to run sometimes and play soccer or basketball other times, or to dance a couple times a week and go bike riding other times.

Include free play if exercise is all structured. School-age kids should get an hour of free play and an hour of good exercise—that's two hours unless the free play is moderate to vigorous exercise.

Don't be too hard on yourself if you can't hit the ideals—some exercise for your child is better than none. A few ideas from parents who have been there can be found in the box on the facing page.

IDEAS FOR MEETING THE EXERCISE CHALLENGE

For many families, fitting in exercise is a real challenge, depending on climate, weather, cost, and neighborhood. It may prove necessary to have different activities in summer and winter. While organized school or community sports after school work for many families, they aren't for all. Here are some examples of other solutions families found:

- Alison went for a long bike ride with her son before school on nice days.
- Alejandro enrolled his daughter in a special martial arts class for children with ADHD.
- Mike installed a heavy punching bag in the basement and taught his teen son how to do workouts with it.
- Jill was able to get her two children outside to jump rope, play hopscotch, play tag, and engage in other active play with some neighbor friends several times a week, enough to see some change in their mood.
- Tania was able to get her daughter into dance lessons that she enjoyed.
- Bob loved running and got his preteen kids interested in going running with him, setting up fun competitions. This resulted in the kids joining running sports in high school as a major hobby.

Sleep and ADHD

Sleep and ADHD are definitely intertwined. Knowledge here has continued to expand rapidly. This is a major lifestyle consideration that goes along with exercise and diet. The science has a lot to tell us about sleep and brain development, as well as about ADHD. It turns out that many children have sleep problems of one sort or another, that sleep's importance is difficult to overestimate, and that many tools are available to boost your child's self-regulation and brain development with better sleep.

Chances are you don't get enough sleep and neither do your kids. National surveys indicate that 70 percent of teens and 70 percent of adults are not getting enough sleep.

First, if you are worried about your child's sleep, you are not alone.

Sleep problems are very common in children. In one recent national survey, over half of parents reported their child had some sort of sleep problem, and *one-fourth* of parents reported their child did not get enough sleep. Based on the prevalence of sleep issues, some of the co-occurrence of ADHD and sleep problems is just the random overlap of two common problems. But let's dig deeper. There are causal connections.

> *Kids use sleep to lock in that day's learning.*

During sleep, the brain grows new connections, stores memories, and repairs cells. One striking scientific finding is called sleep-dependent memory consolidation, or *sleep-dependent learning.* This means it's during sleep that learning takes hold. You may be all too familiar with the common complaint in ADHD that a child seems to learn something one day but then has to learn it all over again the next day. This is an example of failure of memory consolidation. The fact is that children can't learn things if they don't sleep! Sleep is also crucial to managing stress and emotions and having the mental capacity for focused attention, as discussed in Chapter 1 and later when we focus on stress itself in Chapter 7.

As the brain is developing, it uses sleep in different distinct ways in early life. Infants use sleep to generalize from one experience to another. Their naps play a crucial role in learning. Recent experi-

> *Sleep seems to be nature's number-one tool for growing a child's brain.*

ments have shown that babies exposed to new learning remember it if they have napped in between the tests, but not if they stayed awake. Preschoolers use sleep to retain specific things they learned during the day. Children, teens, and adults continue to use sleep to lock in learning.

In recent years, studies like those just mentioned have clarified, in animals and humans, that children and adults learn just as much asleep as while awake. As with babies, when they see new information, they remember it better if they sleep before the memory test than if they don't. Brain-imaging studies using magnetic resonance imaging (MRI) detect patterns of brain activation that show something remarkable: a particular brain pattern activates when seeing new information awake, *and the same pattern is replayed during sleep.* This indicates that during sleep the brain works to consolidate and store what it learned in the daytime.

Now sleep scientists do not see sleep as merely helpful in child learn-

MYTH: NOTHING IMPORTANT HAPPENS DURING SLEEP

Sleep-dependent learning involves the hippocampus, a structure exquisitely organized for different stages of learning and then sending that information to storage. It connects to the frontal cortex to capture new learning and to find out what to retrieve for use in an immediate situation. These brain regions and connections talk to each other and build new wires extensively during childhood—*doing much of their work during sleep.* During sleep they become flexible and able to rewire, and especially in deep sleep, the brain rewires to store new learning. In just the last few years, scientists have been able to show that this process of learning and memory consolidation works in a different way at different stages of development—infancy, childhood, the teen years.

ing—they see it as *necessary.* In fact, some recent studies suggest that children who sleep more have higher IQs, as well as better attention and self-control—all very relevant if your child has ADHD!

SLEEP AND EPIGENETICS

By now you should not be surprised to find out that sleep regulation, like so many other functions, depends not just on genetics but on epigenetic signaling. For example, a study in 2015 looked at pairs of identical twins in which one twin wanted to go to sleep early in the evening and the other wanted to go to sleep later. The study found the twins had differences in epigenetic marks on certain circadian genes—implying changes in how those genes were functioning in the brain. This finding fell right in line with what our group found when we published the first study of the entire epigenome of children with ADHD in 2015. This was a pilot study, meaning it was designed to test out the procedure for a future study, and we are now following up with that much larger study. The preliminary study, meanwhile, identified a handful of genes that showed epigenetic alterations in ADHD in the children with ADHD versus typically developing young people. One of the most prominent was a gene called VIPR2, which is involved in circadian clock regulation. While not confirmed, that finding does raise interesting linkages.

Some sleep problems likely develop from early experiences that disrupt the settings of the brain's circadian clock via epigenetic change. We already know from a great deal of research that the day–night cycle sets off light-sensitive reactions in key areas of babies' brains that are part of their normal development, so babies adapt to the light–dark cycle where they live. Epigenetic changes do that coding in their young brain. If epigenetic changes early in a child's life can affect how the child sleeps, can we provide training or other experiences that will reverse a current sleep problem? We don't know for sure, but everything we've learned so far about epigenetics suggests that it's possible. Let's look at the best ideas for how to resolve a sleep problem.

SLEEP, ATTENTION, AND SELF-REGULATION

We don't need research studies to tell us that we can't focus, pay attention, or concentrate well without good sleep. But science adds an important detail: this problem with attention can carry over even after sleep is restored. You also know from experience that your self-control quickly stumbles after a sleepless night. You can't cope nearly as well with stress, handle your emotions, or focus when overtired. The same goes in spades for kids, of course. In short, if your child isn't getting enough sleep, her attention and behavior may look a lot like ADHD. And what if your child *has* ADHD? Here are the facts regarding sleep and ADHD to keep in mind:

- Sleep is active, not passive. It's an essential part of wiring the brain and learning. Kids with ADHD usually have either delays or losses of brain development, as well as problems learning, so this is fundamental for them to try to recover.

- Lack of sleep can cause symptoms that resemble ADHD because sleep is necessary to maintain the mental capacity needed for self-regulation. Before we diagnose or treat ADHD, we need to make sure sleep is adequate.

- Children with ADHD only *occasionally* have intrinsic sleep disorders (like obstructive sleep apnea or restless legs syndrome). This should be evaluated when management of sleep-related behaviors proves ineffective and your child still shows signs of not being rested.

- Children with ADHD *often* have sleep-related behavior problems that interfere with getting adequate sleep. We'll talk about the difference in a minute.

If your child isn't getting enough sleep, or enough good-quality sleep, then you can expect inattention, disorganization, moodiness, tantrums, irritability, and health problems from more colds to vague complaints. What's worse, your child's brain growth will not be happening under its preferred conditions. If you are like most parents, chances are decent that your kids may not be getting adequate sleep, simply by the law of averages—a substantial percentage of children (and adults) do not get adequate sleep in the United States! Our lives are often just too over-loaded. Once again, many children may be able to tolerate this state of affairs without obvious ill effects. But if your child has ADHD, you have less margin for error to "let this one go." Sleep is an area where it might make a lot of sense to take some action.

HOW MUCH SLEEP SHOULD YOUR CHILD BE GETTING?

How much sleep developing children need may surprise you. The National Sleep Foundation recommends that from zero to two years of age infants and toddlers get more than twelve hours of sleep a day. Many, of course, get some of this by napping. Preschoolers need ten to thirteen hours (for a median of eleven hours). School-age children typi-cally should be getting ten hours of sleep a night (some guidelines suggest eleven hours). While there can certainly be individuals who go outside of these ranges, for most of you that means if your child has to get up at 7:00 for school, she should be asleep by 9:00 P.M., starting to get ready for bed by 8:30 P.M., and turning off screens and ending stimulating activities by 8:00. Teens need only a little less—nine to ten hours, depending on which guidelines one follows. With school starting at 8:00 or 8:30, early bedtimes are required.

This is very difficult for teenagers, whose biological clocks are set for a later cycle than adults by evolution. That change in their body clocks is not an aberration but a normal developmental phase of adolescence. The box below gives some sample sleep schedules based on National Sleep Foundation guidelines (*http://sleepfoundation.org*).

Sleep and Teenagers

The teen years are a special challenge for parents today. Teens are busy—too busy to get the sleep they need, just like adults! They still need at least nine hours of sleep, and ten might be better. Yet only 30 percent of teens even get eight hours of sleep per night. The challenge is particularly serious because teens naturally have later circadian clocks—they don't want to go to bed as early as adults do. Evolution has designed us that way. Ideally, teens could stay up late and sleep late—as many do in the summer and on weekends. This is natural for their development. If your teen has ADHD, however, this creates a difficult situation, because children with ADHD especially can ill afford to lose sleep. A further challenge for everyone is that school schedules conflict with the natural sleep cycle and circadian rhythm for children, and even more for teens. Teens are shoehorned into an early-morning schedule. Our academic calendar

---

HOW MUCH SLEEP DOES MY CHILD NEED?

SAMPLE SCHEDULES

	Target range	Median	Bedtime	Asleep	Wake
Preschool (3–5)	10–13 hrs.	11.5 hrs.	7:00 P.M.	7:30 P.M.	7:00 A.M.
School age (6–13)	9–11 hrs.	10 hrs.	8:30 P.M.	9:00 P.M.	7:00 A.M.
Teen (14–17)	8–10 hrs.	9 hrs.	9:30 P.M.	10:00 P.M.	7:00 A.M.
Young adult (18+)	7–9 hrs.	8 hrs.	10:30 P.M.	11:00 P.M.	7:00 A.M.

makes it harder for teens to get enough sleep. In 2014 the American Academy of Pediatrics issued a policy statement recommending that middle and high school should not start before 8:30 A.M. Yet fewer than 20 percent of schools comply with this recommendation at present; the average start time nationwide is 8:00 A.M., and some start earlier. In 2015 the calls for change grew louder. An expert summary of the problem and recommendations were provided in November 2015 in *Perspectives in Psychological Science,* which recommends pushing back high school start times as late as possible. Some municipalities are actively moving in that direction, and some states have moved most of their schools to an 8:30 or later start.

In the meantime, it's normal for teens, unfortunately, to struggle to go to sleep at night and get up in the morning. For some teens this pattern does cross the line to a delayed sleep–wake phase disorder—but you need a doctor to determine if it has. According to the American Academy of Sleep Medicine, the hallmarks of a delayed sleep–wake phase disorder are (1) difficulty getting to sleep and waking up and (2) sleepiness during the day.

What's Causing the Problem?

If you know your child isn't getting enough sleep and is showing the negative effects of undersleeping, you obviously need to figure out why this is happening. For kids with ADHD, sleep problems fall into two classes:

- Secondary sleep problems, such as problems with bedtime. Here, the problem is usually that ADHD is causing sleep problems!

- Primary sleep problems, such as biological sleep–wake cycle problem or obstructive sleep apnea. Here the sleep problems may be causing ADHD-like symptoms and behavior such as poor concentration, low energy, and irritability. Of course, some children have both types of problems and have ADHD.

Researchers have three basic methods for studying sleep in children, listed in the box on the next page. You can pursue one of these with a professional, but if you think your child has a sleep problem, my recom-

HOW SLEEP PROBLEMS ARE ASSESSED BY A PROFESSIONAL

- A short questionnaire (one is called the Children's Sleep Habits Questionnaire) or a sleep diary.

- A small motion sensor the size of a watch that is worn on the wrist or ankle. It tracks nighttime or twenty-four-hour activity and provides a rough gauge as to when a child is asleep.

- Polysomnography—that is, an overnight sleep study in a lab where the child is attached to electrodes that monitor sleep quality (brain waves) and breathing and other measures directly. This is the "gold standard" but expensive, and only sometimes warranted.

- Additional methods of sleep tracking using sensors and smartphones are emerging but not yet very dependable for clinical purposes. Use these with caution with children due to concerns about effects of blue screens on sleep, which we'll talk about shortly.

mendation is to start simple and just look at bedtime routines and sleep hygiene and attack the problem behaviorally. If the following remedies for secondary sleep problems don't help, that's the time to go further with clinical evaluation and treatment.

Secondary Sleep Problems: Bedtime and Sleep Hygiene

Knowing your child's ideal sleep schedule is the easy part. Creating a calm, successful bedtime routine is a lot more challenging for most parents. If you have a child with ADHD, he may be particularly resistant to bedtime, and because he's tired he may escalate and get a tantrum going right when you are trying to bring the day to a quiet end—and you're tired too! You have stuff to do. It can be very frustrating.

Here are the most common *behavioral sleep problems* recognized by the American Academy of Sleep Medicine. Although these problems are not indicators of ADHD, they are more common in children with the condition. So especially if your child has ADHD, you may recognize some of these.

- Falling asleep is an extended process that requires special conditions.

- Sleep-onset associations are highly problematic or demanding—that is, the child doesn't like to go to sleep.

- Without her special conditions, the child takes a long time to go to sleep or has other sleep disruptions.

- Nighttime awakenings require caregiver intervention for the child to return to sleep.

- Limit-setting problems occur:
  - The child has difficulty initiating or maintaining sleep.
  - The child stalls or refuses to go to bed at an appropriate time.
  - The child refuses to return to bed following a nighttime awakening.

The first line of defense to either prevent or overcome these types of problems is to establish basic "sleep hygiene"—the behavioral routine that makes sleep easier, including the bedtime routine. Let's go over that first.

The core of a good sleep hygiene routine is to have time before bed to prepare the body for sleep. This means that for at least an hour before bedtime your child should avoid blue light (computer, TV, and device screens—next section), large meals, and exercise. That's the time boundary. There is also a space boundary: Keep the bed only for sleeping. (For adults it is advised to keep the whole bedroom only for sleep, but for most families this isn't possible for children, whose bedrooms often double as playrooms and study rooms. But try to keep the *bed* for sleep only.) And as you probably know, it really is a bad idea to keep a TV in the bedroom.

Bottom line: Blue screens are a threat to sleep quality and should be avoided for at least an hour before bed. This includes mobile phones.

Behavioral Approaches to Fixing Sleep Problems. The behavioral sleep problems listed above can occur in any child but seem to be practically epidemic in children with ADHD. They are often caused by the

FAQ: IS THE CELL PHONE OR IPAD CAUSING MY CHILD'S SLEEP PROBLEMS?

Kids with ADHD love their electronics—video games, cell phones, computers, tablets, and TV. One speculation about why they like these things so much is that the frequent changes in stimulation probably help keep dopamine active in the brain and help them maintain an alert state. Unfortunately, these devices are also distracting and can interfere with social development, as I review in Chapter 5. Here there's another concern—the "blue light" they emit interferes with sleep.

Several studies in 2014 and 2015 confirmed what many clinicians long suspected. Children and adults who use mobile phones, computers, or televisions before going to bed sleep more poorly. The body naturally begins to produce melatonin when daylight dims to prepare for sleep. We now know that the blue light of backlit electronic screens is just the right wavelength to suppress that melatonin production. Studies using hourly saliva samples in children and adults confirm dramatic suppression of melatonin when light from the screens is reaching the eyes. Other studies using randomized controlled designs confirm that electronic screen use in the hour before bed causes insomnia (harder to fall asleep), changes in sleep stages (such as REM sleep), and less alertness the next day.

For example, in 2015 researchers in Boston reported striking findings about using e-readers or iPads (or similar devices) compared to reading a print book during the last hour before bed. Those who used the electronic reader were less sleepy, took longer to fall asleep, had later circadian timing (including changes in melatonin and changes in REM sleep), and were less alert the next morning. Those were young adults. The same is now observed in children using a simple correlational design. In 2015, a different group (also in Boston) surveyed over 2,000 fourth- and seventh-graders. Children who slept near a small screen (including sleeping near their phone), played computer games in the evening, or had TV in their room had less sleep and felt less rested. If you're interested in reading the study reports, here are the references to look up:

Chang, A. M., Aeschbach, D., Duffy, J. F., & Czeisler, C. A. (2015). Evening use of light-emitting eReaders negatively affects sleep, circadian timing, and next-morning alertness. *Proceedings of the National Academy of Sciences, 112,* 1232–1237.

Falbe, J., Davison, K. K., Franckle, R. L., Ganter, C., Gortmaker, S. L., Smith, L., et al. (2015). Sleep duration, restfulness, and screens in the sleep environment. *Pediatrics, 135*(2)., e367–375.

child having negative mental associations with going to bed or going to sleep. So one key concept is to replace those associations over time with very positive ones—making bedtime a really rewarding experience for the child.

Most parents are familiar with various sleep training programs and a welter of different advice for getting their babies on a regular sleep schedule. Even for school-age kids, however, a "sleep training" program is a helpful concept, even if the application is a little different than with infants. If your child has ADHD, then this type of approach may be particularly helpful in overcoming a sleep/bedtime behavior problem.

A randomized controlled clinical trial in 2014 showed that a formal "sleep training program"—that is, a professionally guided behavior program with a counselor—led to noticeable improvements in mood, emotion, and overall adjustment for children with ADHD. In comparison, simply giving parents information about sleep hygiene did not fare as well. The reason is probably obvious to you—implementing a new sleep schedule is not easy, and you may need a consistent, carefully designed behavior management program to make it work. See the action steps on the next page for the basics, but note that you may need to get a pro to

---

WHEN YOU NEED HELP WITH BEHAVIORAL SLEEP DIFFICULTIES

Behavioral sleep difficulties often don't clear up on their own. When they go on for a long time, there is a significant danger that they'll become entrenched. Professional counselors can help you choose from among a number of possible formal behavioral training programs. These include:

- positive routines
- unmodified extinction
- graduated extinction
- extinction with parental presence

They all work about equally well so you can work with a psychologist or counselor trained in behavioral medicine to choose the one you want to try and set up a formal program. You can start by trying to set up a program of your own, following the action steps on page 110; then, if that doesn't improve matters, get professional guidance.

guide you through setting it up and troubleshooting. The good news: the counseling need not be very intensive. Another recent study found improvement after parents received just two sessions of expert guidance on getting a behavioral sleep program in place.

 AT A GLANCE

Action Steps for Good Sleep Hygiene

Basics

- No TV in the bedroom.
- Turn off and remove blue light (all screens including cell phones) for at least an hour before bedtime; no use of cell phones in the bed.
- Avoid large meals right before bedtime.
- Keep the bedroom, or at least the bed, only for sleeping; study elsewhere.
- No vigorous exercise for at least an hour before bed; keep things calm and low key.
- Set up a routine that takes 30–45 minutes.
- Keep the child moving forward during the routine; redirect as necessary.
- Conclude with a very positive ritual enjoyable to the child (for example, a story or song together).
- End the routine with good night and the child in bed alone, drowsy but awake (so he doesn't think he needs you present to fall asleep the rest of the way).

Tips

- If the child calls you back or leaves the room, minimize engagement and redirect to sleep.
- Maintain total consistency, with the same routine and schedule every night.
- The best rewards are praise and affection—keep it positive.

- But use points if you have to in order to keep the child motivated to follow the routine.
- Write out the schedule if that helps the child target what you want.
- Counselors can help you create a stronger, more formal behavioral plan if needed.

FAQ: IS ADHD MEDICATION CAUSING MY CHILD TO HAVE SLEEP PROBLEMS?

A systematic review of the literature in 2015 evaluated this question. While it was disappointing how few high-quality studies have really been conducted (only nine studies on 246 children—meaning one large study could overturn the result), important interim conclusions nonetheless emerged. It appears that prescriptions of stimulant medication are associated with a greater chance of

- later sleep onset (child takes longer to fall asleep). Indeed, some reviews find that 25–50 percent of children with ADHD have some type of problem with getting to sleep on time.
- shorter sleep duration—kids get less sleep.
- reduced sleep quality (evaluated by overnight studies with electrical sensors to measure respiration, sleep stage, and other variables).

For children who must take stimulants, certain factors reduced these problems. First, the longer a child was on stimulants, the more her body adjusted and sleep got closer to normal. Thus, monitor sleep but give it a few weeks to see if your child's body adjusts back to normal sleep.

Second, the dosing schedule made a difference. It may help to ask your doctor to try a different dosing schedule, medication at a different time of day, or skipping an evening dose. Alternatively, instead of a long-acting or timed-release preparation, use a traditional short-acting compound to see if that removes the sleep interference effect.

When stimulants like Concerta or Adderall are prescribed, sleep should be tracked. This can be done by filling out a simple sleep diary or sleep log for a period of time (examples are easily found online at the National Sleep Foundation website, for example, *https://sleepfoundation.org/ sleep-diary/SleepDiaryv6.pdf*).

Primary Sleep Disorders and ADHD

In addition to getting on a good sleep schedule and practicing good sleep hygiene to address the behavioral side of sleep, sleep itself has to be good quality. Poor sleep habits like watching TV before bed can cause insomnia as well as poor quality of sleep when sleeping. However, insomnia or poor sleep quality can also be caused by a primary sleep disorder related to something biological. If the behavioral steps just covered aren't cutting it, or if your child has the warning signs mentioned below, then a sleep specialist consultation is a good idea.

In 2015 researchers looking at ADHD and sleep completed a pooled analysis of studies using motion sensors on wrists and ankles to evaluate sleep. They identified twenty-four relevant studies involving over 2,100 children. That review showed that in fact children with ADHD on average do have worse sleep, with less time in deep sleep. Some of these problems will be a primary sleep disorder. While the motion sensors give a good indication something is wrong, the gold standard is *polysomnography* (studies in sleep labs), mentioned earlier. Because polysomnography studies are costly, generalizable studies are few. But the picture from what we do have still is notable. *While most kids with ADHD have behavioral sleep issues, such as not getting to bed on time, only a small percentage have true primary sleep disorders.* Still, it's important to know about these if your child has ADHD.

Delayed Sleep–Wake Phase Syndrome. Among the primary sleep disorders, the most common, and the one that is raising the most concern in relation to ADHD in the current science, is this one (formerly called *delayed sleep phase syndrome*). Ask your doctor if you suspect this problem. (Most of the time the doctor can make the diagnosis by interview and exam. In rare instances the doctor may want to obtain saliva samples to measure melatonin production.) The solution may be as simple as a revised schedule to help your child's body realign with the light cycle or another behavioral program. In other cases, a melatonin supplement may be helpful (see the box on the facing page). As mentioned earlier, professional help is necessary to diagnose this, particularly with adolescents, for whom evolution has already pushed the sleep–wake phase far out of sync with our modern school schedules, making diagnosis more difficult. That said, here are the signs you can watch for:

FAQ: SHOULD I TRY MELATONIN FOR MY CHILD WITH ADHD?

What Is Melatonin? Melatonin is a hormone that regulates the daily circadian (wake–sleep) cycle. The body makes more melatonin when it gets dark to prepare us to sleep, and less when it gets light to prepare us to be awake. Melatonin is widely used to help adults with insomnia. It is a hormone, so even though it is sold over the counter, side effect risks are real.

Guidance. Use melatonin with your child only under medical supervision and after a behavioral program fails. Based on the proceedings of a consensus conference of experts in 2014, melatonin, properly dosed, can be safe and effective to help children fall asleep (shorter "sleep latency") and sleep longer. However, it does not reduce nighttime awakenings—it helps kids fall asleep but not *stay* asleep. Genetic variation in how they metabolize melatonin leads to better effects at lower doses for some people. Note that many over-the-counter tablets provide far too high a dose for children.

Does It Help ADHD? In the case of ADHD, the consensus conference identified only three randomized trials; each showed a benefit to sleep onset but *not* to ADHD symptoms during the day.

Risks. We have insufficient knowledge of the risks of long-term melatonin supplements for children's still-developing endocrine system. Concerns about affecting your child's development are particularly notable with infants (their bodies are still learning how to adjust sleep and melatonin to local light cycles) and teens (whose bodies are working with rapidly changing hormone levels already).

Side Effects. Though not usual, side effects can include waking up in the middle of the night, a morning "hangover" (feeling drowsy, headache, feeling "down"), daytime laziness, excessive sweating at night or in the day, and bedwetting.

Bottom Line. Melatonin can be a useful way to help restore your child to a normal sleep cycle, especially if he is diagnosed with sleep–wake phase disorder and behavior adjustments have not worked. But poor sleep hygiene, depression, or health problems can mimic a sleep–wake phase disorder, so fix sleep hygiene and get a health checkup with your pediatrician first. Because melatonin is a hormone and its interactions with normal hormone changes in developing children are not well understood, work with your doctor.

WANT TO READ MORE?

For the 2014 consensus conference report, see the following article:

Bruni, O., Alonso-Alconada, D., Besag, F., Biran, V., Braam, W., Cortese, S., et al. (2015). Current role of melatonin in pediatric neurology: Clinical recommendations. *European Journal of Paediatric Neurology, 19*(2), 122–133.

- Not being sleepy at night
- Not being able to fall asleep at bedtime
- Struggling to wake up in the morning
- Sometimes tired or sleepy during the day (or naps or sleeps easily during the day)

Other Primary Sleep Disorders. The other common disorders include *obstructive sleep apnea* and *periodic limb movements*. Obstructive apnea is more likely in individuals who are overweight. Periodic limb movements occur often in children with *restless legs syndrome*; iron deficiency can contribute to restless legs syndrome and periodic limb movements. For an individual child, the only definite way to identify a primary sleep problem is polysomnography.

Warning Signs of a Primary Sleep Disorder. Warning signs are not diagnostic, but they can help you decide whether your child might need a professional sleep evaluation. Watch for these signs in your child:

- Snores frequently even when not sick.
- Bedcovers frequently end up on the floor—even when it's cold.
- Is hanging half off the bed while sleeping (suggesting a lot of restless movement in sleep).
- Sleepwalks or has night terrors (wakes up screaming) more than once or twice.
- Can't wake up or resists getting up despite enough (apparent) sleep.

  TAKE-HOME POINTS

Sleep and ADHD

- Blue screens interfere with sleep; limiting them helps sleep and creates more time for free play and exercise.
- Try to improve your child's sleep hygiene behaviorally first; that may do the trick for your child. Excellent self-help resources are

available online from the National Sleep Foundation (*https://sleepfoundation.org*).

- If you are struggling to get your child's bedtime-related behavior into a positive place or suspect a sleep disorder, seek a professional evaluation.

Keep in mind that a healthy lifestyle is synergistic. It helps all children and helps physical and emotional health. If your child has ADHD, your reduced margin for error means these are very attractive options to take advantage of. And each action step you decide to take is likely to boost the effects of the others. As noted in the take-home points for exercise, a good diet provides more fuel for exercising. So too, exercise and sleep are a virtuous cycle—one promotes the other. As you read through this book, think about what seems likely to help your child most, as well as what will be most practical for your family. The last chapter in the book will give you a chance to review all these ideas and choose the scientifically sound tools that will work for your child.

5

Technology and ADHD

Latest Findings on the Peril and the Promise

What's the latest understanding of technology and ADHD? This may be the most common question parents ask. On the one hand, computer technology seems to be a real challenge. Kids with ADHD love their screens. Aside from what we covered on blue screens and sleep in Chapter 4, can use of screens, video games, or TV actually cause ADHD or make it worse? The answer is complex. The big news is that secondary problems like aggression are definitely made worse by watching violent media. Yet direct effects of media usage on ADHD symptoms, while likely real, are slight. Meanwhile, kids with ADHD are at secondary risk from Internet use that parents should understand and can, with understanding, protect them from.

At the same time, recent years have seen an explosion of new high-tech efforts to diagnose and treat mental health, neurological, and cognitive disorders using computers. The diagnostic promise is significant. New diagnostic methods enable a computer to draw from thousands of potential questions and in a matter of minutes, asking just a handful of questions, arrive at the same conclusion as a much longer and more detailed interview. This represents real progress, raising the possibility that within a few years more clinicians will be able to evaluate and diagnose neurodevelopmental problems like ADHD faster and more accurately, meaning concerns will be addressed earlier and kids will get the help they need more quickly. Other diagnostic technologies, such as brain imaging methods, are not yet ready for prime time, as outlined below.

In the case of treatment, however, the situation is still ambiguous. In some cases, new high-tech treatments may provide powerful new avenues for potentially treating neurological and psychiatric problems. The days of crude, intrusive brain alterations are gone; we are looking at a future filled with wide-ranging electronics designed to affect and improve brain function. Because these newer tools are costly and don't offer the intrinsic general health benefits of a good diet or exercise or sufficient sleep, however, we have to raise the bar for proof that they are effective before suggesting you try them for your child with ADHD. While I will advise you to bypass computerized and electronic treatment approaches for now, it's important to acquaint yourself with them and with the status of the science on them. This knowledge will equip you to critically monitor new developments that are surely on their way and could change these conclusions. We'll cover the following "hot topics" that you may have seen on TV or in the newspaper or in your own Internet searches for breakthrough assessment and treatment:

- Computerized cognitive training of attention (for example, Cog-med)
- Neurofeedback (aka biofeedback), both active and passive
- Direct brain stimulation (transcranial magnetic or direct-current stimulation)

But first let's get to the bottom of the complex relationship of electronic screen use and ADHD.

Screen Time and ADHD: Sifting Fact from Fiction

I've already noted (in Chapter 4) that too much screen time, especially in the evening, can cause sleep problems due to the blue light entering the eyes. But what about TV, games, or other screens somehow causing ADHD? Here we have a combination of

1. Direct-effect questions: Can watching too much TV weaken the development of attention or cause related problems associated with ADHD?

2. Indirect-effect questions: How does ADHD make kids more vulnerable to potentially negative consequences of using electronics?

Whether media use or exposure can cause ADHD is a very common concern. Again, the biggest story here is related to ADHD secondarily: science has established that violent content in games and TV shows can make aggressive tendencies worse, and aggressive tendencies are a major concern for kids with ADHD due to their weaker self-regulation (see the box on the facing page). The news about whether media use affects ADHD, attention, and self-regulation is less earth-shaking: too much media does weaken attention and add to ADHD, but only slightly. Questions of direct causation aside, perhaps the biggest concern for parents of children with ADHD is often how much their kids are using, or want to use, electronic media. Many note an "addictive" tendency of kids with ADHD toward technology, although that claim is short on scientific proof. Regardless, given the social hazards of the Internet, many parents worry because their children seem so determined to use media as much as possible.

OPPORTUNITY OR RISK?

The informational and educational potential of today's electronic devices is mind-boggling. The pros and cons are complex. On the one hand, using these computerized tools may help kids learn about technology. This idea tempts many parents to get their toddler an iPad. The technology is also invading school classrooms, touted as a learning aid. Tools like iPads, screen media, and even video games can have positive educational value. Some games teach kids how to read; others can help them learn math. At the same time, we have to admit these games are not all so good. Meanwhile, kids are lost in their screens too, and this worries many parents. At times, it seems all too easy to blame all of society's ills

ADHD AND RISK FOR AGGRESSION

While this is not new, it's important to realize that for kids with hyperactive/impulsive behavior problems serious enough to meet criteria for ADHD, one of the major downstream risks is emergence of aggressive antisocial behavior. Some 50 percent of children with ADHD develop serious sustained problems in this area—way above the average for other kids (less than 5 percent, not counting a burst of antisocial behavior that sometimes emerges for a short time in the teenage years). As with all things about ADHD, this is only a subgroup of kids with ADHD. Warning signs include:

- Being flagrantly defiant of adults (flat-out refusing to obey teachers and parents)

- Indifference to punishment or seeming unconcern with what will happen

- Blaming others all the time for their feelings or problems (not counting just their sibling)

- Teachers or other parents complaining they are too domineering, bossy, or aggressive

- School reports of fighting

- Being extremely angry much of the time

If your child shows even some of these behaviors more than rarely, this is a warning sign. Although toddlers are "aggressive" (such as pushing another toddler to get their toy), they outgrow this with normal development. Aggression in older children tends to be a learned behavior in that earlier aggression gets modeled or encouraged somehow. It can be learned at home (for example, through constant mutually threatening exchanges between parents and kids) or from peers (through modeling and other effects) and from social media (Internet, television). Recent meta-analysis has confirmed that watching violent media content increases hostile thoughts and interpretations of social situations. Some kids with ADHD are vulnerable to going down this road because of their weakness in social learning (that is, not picking up on expected social norms as readily as other children). This means they are more vulnerable to explicit demonstrations of aggressive behavior as something to copy or to try.

on screen media. It is also tempting to let the video game, the TV, or the computer do the babysitting. "My son gets absorbed, and I can do other stuff! I'm happy; he's happy: seems like a win-win!" For some families, there's not much choice because there is just too much going on.

For example, Joe and Candace shared with me during an evaluation that they have two special-needs school-age boys—one with severe ADHD, the other with a physical disability—and an infant. While both parents work long hours at their low-wage jobs, the kids are difficult to manage. The only way to get any control seems to be to let them sit in front of a computer game or movie a lot of the time. But Joe and Candace naturally wonder how this is affecting the boys' development and their son's ADHD symptoms. What the various gadgets and tools can do is constantly changing, and of course new hardware and new platforms readily pop onto the scene. At the moment, technological devices that kids often have access to include:

- Computers
- Video game players
- Television (now with Internet-based on-demand movies and shows)
- Notebooks and tablets
- Cell phones
- Portable music players
- Internet-connected watches

By the time you're reading this book, this list will probably be getting out of date. What you need to know now and going forward is that all of these devices (with the possible exception of watches) have blue-light screens that can interfere with melatonin production and sleep, as noted in Chapter 4. All (even some watches) can access the Internet. Once the user is on the Internet, additional tools are available: social networking sites (such as Facebook); file and picture sharing sites (Snapchat); communication sites (like Twitter); search engines (Google); shopping; video and TV shows (Hulu, Amazon); and chat. Through these media, clearly children get access to extraordinary amounts of information and opportunities to learn and be educated, *if they can manage it all*. For most, that's a big *if*. Common concerns include:

- Distracting, attention-grabbing information that may affect attention and focus
- Violent content that can be distracting or overstimulating, or inspire harmful actions
- Pornographic, explicit, or disturbing sexual content beyond their maturity level
- Disclosure of their personal information to public viewing
- Sexual predators
- Online bullying and harassment
- Ideological extremists (such as terrorist groups)
- So-called comment boards filled with nasty, hostile, or demeaning exchanges

These media are increasingly sophisticated; they comprise the most powerful teaching technologies ever developed. Their frequent yet unpredictable feedback to the user makes them inherently rewarding and habit forming. However, these new tools, which can have true educational and entertainment value (and truly can give parents a much-needed break), also have a dark side when it comes to children's healthy development of executive functioning, self-control, prosocial behavior, and attention. Besides interfering with sleep quality, they compete with exercise, free play, and homework!

Here's the latest science on a couple of the big negatives.

Screen Media, Violent Content, and Aggressive Behavior and ADHD

The most common serious complication for children with ADHD is aggression, as noted earlier. Are screen media contributing to this risk? We now know they are. In fact, scientists have known for quite a long time that unrestricted TV and video games hurt children due to the violence they contain. An hour a day of unrestricted commercial television will mean a child witnesses, in one week, dozens of extreme violent acts (murders, assaults, even rape). This is true in cartoons as well as dramas. Art does *not* "reflect life" here; screen media show a lot more violence than the world really has, giving children a distorted understanding of the social world.

The violence on TV far exceeds the frequency of violence in the real world.

This is not just overload to your child's psyche. The science now shows that it causes more aggressive acting-out behavior both in the short term and over the lifespan. This is one of the most well-established findings in scientific psychology—and one of the least well known. More than a decade ago, the Association for Psychological Science published an authoritative summary in its publication *Psychological Science in the Public Interest*. The scientific evidence here is conclusive, with a large, varied set of hundreds of observational and experimental studies. Comprehensive literature reviews of hundreds of studies have given the same picture.

Bottom line: It's the real deal that TV and game violence increases aggression in children who are susceptible to aggression; kids with ADHD are susceptible to aggression.

Media violence primes the automatic parts of our psyche with scripts, routines, and schemas that involve aggressive behavior. Remember from Chapter 1, *automatic* routines govern most of our behavior and are part of self-regulation. We exert mental control to override them. In the heat of the moment, people who watch more media violence are more prone to activate these automatic aggressive scripts. Not all children are affected equally; some are practically immune to these media effects. However, kids with ADHD are in the group that is not immune— they are often susceptible to this rescripting.

The causal relation between violent screen images and increases in aggressive behavior in a general population sample is similar in strength to that for smoking and lung cancer.

Is this effect really big enough to worry about? Yes. From a public health point of view, the association here is like the importance of aspirin to heart attack or smoking to lung cancer. It's one of the clearest public health associations we know about.

Action Step

It is important to monitor what sort of media your child with ADHD is interacting with. If he is having trouble with aggressive behavior or ideas, restrict what he can watch on TV, video games, or other screen media until he demonstrates he can handle it.

SCREEN MEDIA, ATTENTION DEVELOPMENT, AND ADHD

Less clear has been whether television and video games, due to either their highly arousing nature or their fast-paced, attention-grabbing presentation, weaken the development of attention and executive functioning. A countervailing concern is that by removing children from social interaction, screen media dampen their social and language skills. As intuitively appealing as these ideas may seem, the scientific literature is small, methodologically weak, and ultimately rather inconclusive.

> *There is a **small** association between media use and ADHD symptoms, mainly inattention.*

We can, however, get a glimpse, using our hockey metaphor, of where this puck is going. In 2015, scientists were able to put together the first truly authoritative meta-analysis summary of screen media use and ADHD based on enough studies to be meaningful. The result of this formal analysis was the finding that there is in fact an overall association of more screen media use and more symptoms of ADHD—including a few experimental studies that support a causal linkage. As you might suspect, this is particularly the case for inattention, rather than hyperactivity or impulsivity. However, this association is quite small—certainly smaller than the effect of media on aggression, and also smaller than most other risk factors for ADHD. Whether this average effect masks bigger effects for some children is unknown. It was not clear what might cause the association. Do the screens directly disrupt attention development? Or do they simply keep children from the hands-on engagement with people and things they need to grow their brain fully, and thus *indirectly* interfere with development?

Although this effect is small, success for kids with ADHD means addressing as many obstacles to their development as we can. If you can manage it, put limits on your child's amount of screen time in addition to monitoring the content. Fortunately, if your child is getting an hour of free play, plenty of exercise, doing homework, and going to bed early enough to get ten or eleven hours of sleep, with no screens allowed in the bedroom after hours, there isn't much time left for excessive use of screen media.

 AT A GLANCE

Action Step

Make sure your child gets enough exercise and sleep (see Chapter 4), and there won't be much time left for excessive media use. Consider imposing the limits shown in the box below.

FAQ: WHAT ARE REASONABLE LIMITS FOR MEDIA USE?

From the American Academy of Pediatrics (AAP):

For Average Children and Teenagers. At most one to two hours per day of *high-quality* media time. For a child with ADHD, it will make sense to stay on the low end of this range—sixty to ninety minutes per day maximum. That's challenging, because kids with ADHD seem even more attracted to the easy brain stimulation (and easy "dopamine kick") that video games and other media provide. But it's a good guide. Note the emphasis on *high-quality* time—meaning you are aware of what the child is able to watch or do.

For Toddlers under Two Years of Age. Zero screen media. The Zero to Three association is more lenient: they suggest screen time for toddlers be "limited," carefully monitored, and that parents cement the distinction between screen and real events. This would suggest that any screen media for age two years and under occur only with a parent so you can share the experience, interpret it for the child, and monitor it.

New AAP guidelines are due out about the time this book is published. Watch for those—but I don't expect major changes.

Social Media and Managing Internet Safety: What Works?

Children with ADHD make social mistakes; they misread social cues; and they get into mixed-up social relationships. In this light, a concern for many parents is unrestricted Internet access via all their devices. According to national surveys by the Pew Foundation, as of 2013, 95 percent of American teens had Internet access; 75 percent had a mobile phone or device. By the time you read this, those numbers certainly will be even higher. The main access point for many teens, their mobile phone, has many advantages. But it also privatizes the child's experience and makes it more difficult for parents to monitor what their children are doing online or via social media.

Mobile phone use interferes with attention and focus simply by its distracting nature. We see this with adults who cannot focus during a meeting because they are distracted by an incoming text message. We see it in the scientific findings that a major cause of car accidents is drivers looking at their mobile device. We see it in college students distracted by their phone during a college lecture. We see it in pedestrians walking into traffic while staring at their phone.

But the major concerns for children in the clinical literature (and among parents) are safety risks from the Internet itself: sexual victimization, cyberbullying, harassment, and even the rare but dangerous links to extremist ideologies. Impulsive children with poor self-control are more at risk due to the ease with which the device can capture their attention (novelty, which triggers a dopamine release), impulsive responding, and misjudgment of social context.

How frequently do these problems occur? No one is sure, but the best evidence is that *serious* problems, while common enough to warrant taking precautions, are far from universal—and tragic outcomes are reassuringly rare. Thus, there is reason for prudence and engagement, but not alarm. When they occur, the more serious risks of the Internet are related to *excessive* Internet or mobile usage (that is, much beyond the guidelines in the box on page 124). For example, two large recent studies reported that more mobile Internet use was associated with a greater chance of sexual or other victimization and riskier exposures (pornographic, violent, or extremist content). Other risk factors in the literature are lack of parental monitoring (child secrecy), child lack of awareness of risks, low child self-esteem, and child tendency to break rules.

Bottom line: While not all risky exposures are automatically harmful and the *most tragic* harms are *rare*, parental attention is warranted in monitoring mobile Internet use and taking the active precautions summarized in the box that follows, particularly if you have an impulsive or socially insecure child.

 AT A GLANCE

Action Steps to Reduce Internet Risks for Impulsive Children

- Stay involved and communicate with your children about their online activity.
- Teach online safety: Monitor your children's security settings and public disclosures.
- Ensure child self-esteem.
- Address rule-breaking habits.
- Separate out online gaming and recognize it may have an important peer-connection aspect for some teens. If it does, then teach your child safety rules and make an agreement on reasonable amounts of use so it does not crowd out other important activities and social opportunities.
- If your child cannot stick to an agreement on reasonable use or things are getting out of hand, seek professional advice. A well-considered behavioral plan may be needed (see Chapter 9 for more on those methods).

 TAKE-HOME POINTS

Screen Media, Gaming, and Internet Use

Monitor. Be involved. Be nosy! Whether it is TV and video-game violence or online risks, the best science says a major influence on safety is the degree of parent involvement. With TV and video, spend time watching what your child is watching so you know what it is. With Internet use via computer or mobile phone, be involved enough to know what your children are looking at, encourage them to show you, spend time with them, stay engaged and informed. Balance it out—avoid overintrusiveness, but insist on open communication. As best you can, use explanation and try to build partnership; most of all, don't disengage. Keep at it.

Discuss. Interpret. Some data suggest that when parents talk about and interpret TV, video, and online content with a child, they help the child put it in perspective. Ask questions, be curious, discuss. You can do this without being overly critical about your child's choices, and you can also model this with your own Internet use.

Teach Safety. When it comes to the Internet, safety talk is necessary. Like any powerful tool, the Internet carries serious danger if used improperly by a child. Discuss with and teach your child how to stay safe, how to protect privacy and check security settings, and educate her about the risks and how to avoid them. Set ground rules: Require your children to let you see what they are seeing and posting online and to let you check their security settings.

Limit. More screen time and more online use equals more risk. The more time with violent media, the more influence on automatic behavior routines. Limit screen time. More use is riskier because children who are online for more time are the same ones who have been shown to make excessive personal disclosures (blogging, having a publicly viewable Facebook or social networking profile). Again, this holds especially for children who tend toward risk taking and rule breaking. So monitor amount of use, make sure it is not cutting into other necessary activities (sleep, exercise, and face-to-face social activity), and treat general rule-breaking elsewhere as a red flag regarding Internet risks.

Get to Know Your Child's Friends. Risks go up if your child has few friends, is bullied offline, or has friends who approve of risky behaviors. Conversations with the teacher and contact with your child's friends are prudent steps. Welcome your child's friends to your house so you can get acquainted with them.

Model Appropriate Use. One recent study observed fifty families at home during a meal. They found a solid correlation between parents' being absorbed in the cell phone and children acting out. Monitor your own use and hold yourself to the same standard as your kids.

Be Child-Specific. As outlined in a recent authoritative review by Sonia Livingston and Peter Smith in 2014, various Internet safety programs are not sufficiently individualized to be very effective. Take a thoughtful approach tailored to your particular child, taking into account her developmental level and readiness for opportunities and risks.

Technology and ADHD Treatment

In Chapters 8 and 9 I review the state of the art for ADHD treatment and provide some guidance on balancing traditional or "mainstream" and emerging or "alternative" treatments. Here I focus specifically on some new high-tech treatments that are just emerging. It's important you know about them, even though they aren't yet ready to be part of your master plan. Here's what we know to date about how new technologies can help your child with ADHD symptoms and associated problems.

COMPUTERIZED COGNITIVE TRAINING

What Is It? Computerized cognitive training means your child sits in front of a computer and tries to solve problems it presents. These problems challenge skills like working memory, selective attention, or response inhibition to build up these skills. Newer versions are adaptive, meaning they adjust their difficulty to the child's learning progress. They also are more complex, targeting multiple skills at once. Tests of these newest, more sophisticated computer programs are still forthcoming, but we have a sizable literature on the "first generation" of computer-based attention training for ADHD.

The theory is that new neural growth will be triggered and the brain will improve its overall capacity for self-regulation. The most well known of these methods for ADHD at the moment is called Cogmed, developed in Sweden but now marketed to consumers by Pearson. It has been the best studied in relation to ADHD and therefore is my main focus here. Other, more recent tools are under development. For example, a suite of games developed at UC San Francisco attempts to use a sophisticated gaming format to engage and motivate children and activate relevant brain regions, on the theory that the motivation and engagement is a vital part of the cognitive skill growth. It is not yet in commercial or clinical use. Several other such products are on the market and are in active use for ADHD around the country. Most are not well studied in relation to ADHD, except Cogmed. They are often costly, and the data on their value is mixed or quite preliminary—not enough to cross the threshold for me to recommend them for your child.

Is This a New Idea? No, the basic idea of computerized skill training has been around for decades. It features a good theory—after all, the brain can change with training and learning, and epigenetics tells us permanent changes can be created by appropriate stimulation. The literature has shown that computer programs can effectively help people with specific skills such as reading and possibly with memory. A 2016 meta-analysis concluded that depressed adults get some mood benefit from computerized programs designed to improve mood, although that result was quite tentative due to very small studies and very few good measures. However, for decades, the larger question plaguing scientists has been whether practicing a global capacity like working memory (not targeted on an operational skill like reading) can lead to improvement in other settings or abilities that were not trained. In the case of ADHD, the big question is whether computerized working memory training (for example) can actually improve concentration and performance, or even behavior, in school or at home. Strong claims have been made by those marketing these products that such specialty computer programs or games can do so and can even improve IQ. On balance, however, the data don't justify those conclusions. It seems that improving a skill like attention on a computer just does not generalize to skills like self-control in the classroom.

> Current data don't support claims that computer training translates to improvements at school, home, or anywhere other than the computer training program or closely related activities.

Worryingly for this entire approach of computerized cognitive train-

FAQ: I'VE HEARD OF BRAIN-TRAINING COMPUTER PROGRAMS. ARE THEY A SCAM?

There is serious science behind the best of these computer programs. My lab is even collaborating in a treatment trial for one of the newer games. Scientists like the originator of Cogmed are trying to do it right and, when speaking about their data, are balanced, careful, and admirably transparent about the data (and in the case of Cogmed, the originator has refused any financial benefit from his work). However, the products have been marketed prematurely and oversold, well beyond what the data justifies. ADHD is a relatively new market.

Be aware that computer programs have a much longer, and checkered, history for older adults anxious to prevent cognitive decline with aging. This underscores the risks of overly enthusiastic marketing.

A major meta-analysis in 2014 found small benefits for older adults using computerized cognitive training for verbal memory and processing speed, but not attention or executive function—the domains we care about for ADHD. Further, the focal effects, although small, emerged only via *group* training classes, not in at-home solo computer practice—suggesting the social context was somehow important in the effects that were seen. Finally, real-life functioning and durability of changes were not studied. A large systematic review of at-risk older adults (those starting to have cognitive decline) was more optimistic, concluding there were benefits for this population even on laboratory tests of attention and executive function, but the reviewers noted study quality was poor, samples were small, and real-life benefits were unclear. Furthermore, a major comprehensive summary conducted for the authoritative series *Psychological Science in the Public Interest* in 2016 arrived at the conclusion that effects for children do not generalize beyond tasks and skills closely related to the training task.

> The big question about computer training for children with ADHD is whether any improvements seen during training generalize to the child's daily life. So far, we don't have convincing evidence that they do.

ing, in 2014, dozens of leading neuroscientists signed on to a statement sponsored by the Max Planck Institute for Human Development and the Stanford Center on Longevity. They criticized what they said were exaggerated claims by the computer training industry. Studies supporting these industry claims for their products are often small, poorly controlled, fail to take into account motivation or expectancy effects, and fail to show whether the games are superior to—or even as good as—other healthy life activities like going for a walk or socializing. Their consensus statement noted that these games may improve specific skills on the computer (proving only that we are never too old to learn something new) but do not necessarily generalize well to other situations or global cognitive improvement or brain health. They emphasized that other activities, like exercise, socializing, and maintaining a healthy lifestyle, are a better use of time than most brain games. They pointed to the enduring problem with the idea that a single test or mode of practice (such as a computer) can cause general gains in cognitive skills. Any cognitive challenge (playing chess, doing crossword puzzles, playing Sudoku), whether or not on a computer, can improve focus and memory to some extent and is thought to help protect brain health in aging.

This perspective gives us some caution in approaching the effort to use computerized cognitive training to help children with ADHD. Here we have to ask the following questions:

1. Do computerized training programs simply "teach to the test," or do they generalize to other cognitive abilities or other settings?
2. Do they actually help everyday functioning by improving self-control, improving classroom learning, or improving behavior?
3. Most of all, are they more effective than alternative activities like exercise?

The bottom line is (1) they mostly teach to the test, (2) if so, not by much, and (3) unknown but doubtful.

Computerized Cognitive Training and ADHD. For ADHD, several major computerized training programs are now on the market. They have had mixed reviews. A special issue of the *Child and Adolescent Psychiatric Clinics of North America* in late 2014 provided an authoritative summary. The same scientists published a more detailed meta-analytic analysis in another journal a few months later in 2015. Those reviews were able to identify just over a dozen randomized controlled trials (that is, studies with potential to provide causal evidence). The conclusions were somewhat nuanced but can be summarized as follows:

- Parents, who were probably *not* "blind" to the intervention, saw a modest improvement in symptoms of inattention.
- Working memory and tests in the laboratory showed small improvement.
- Clearly blinded raters (such as teachers) did not see reliable changes in ADHD symptoms.
- There was no reliable gain in academic performance.
- Programs that challenge multiple functions (not just working memory, for example) did better than those that did not, but still did not cross the "generalizability" barrier.
- Overall, computerized cognitive training is not (yet?) an effective treatment for ADHD. It may prove helpful in targeted areas such as math or reading or in some settings.

  TAKE-HOME POINTS

Computer Training

It will be difficult to show enduring, generalizable change on ADHD symptoms or classroom behavior by using a computerized cognitive training program—even one that blends sophisticated multitasking and motivational elements (the best will soon do this, so we'll find out).

Be very cautious before spending money on computerized training programs for your child. These programs can be expensive, so the bar should be high for evidence. Such programs may serve as a backup to help some kids with memory skills or reading, or to supplement other specific learning targets, but their ADHD benefit is doubtful. If future studies do reach the ability to show a reliable effect, this type of treatment likely will be an adjunct to other treatments, not an ADHD cure.

Most important, other health activities can be done instead of spending precious free time on computer training; as we've seen, activities like exercise have far better evidence of benefits.

In summary, given the costs of these programs, their controversial marketing at times, and the weak results from expert reviews, I cannot recommend them for your child with ADHD. I strongly hope that picture will look brighter in a few years, but to return to our hockey metaphor: this is a case where the puck may *not* be going there. These treatments warrant continued study because the potential value is great; but there is a real likelihood that they will remain in a niche position.

EEG BIOFEEDBACK (NEUROFEEDBACK) AND ADHD

What Is It? In traditional biofeedback, a machine shows you your heart rate, or blood pressure, and you change your mental state to improve the values. People can learn to do this, and it can be effective in areas like stress reduction, hypertension, and smoking cessation. The concept for ADHD is analogous, only using the brain instead of the heart to try to correct the brain-wave pattern assumed to be off track in ADHD. A machine records your brain waves, and you watch a corresponding display on a computer screen and learn to change the display by changing your mental state. I mentioned in Chapter 1 the idea that ADHD is related to cortical underarousal as seen in excess slow-wave activity. Neurofeedback uses a biofeedback system to try to correct this, to teach a child to alter his brain arousal (brain waves) to a more optimal mix for effective attention.

In a typical task, the child sits in front of a computer with electrodes on his scalp (typically embedded in a cap like a swimmer's cap) and, using only his thoughts, tries to hold a red ball in the center of the circle or does some similar task that affects his brain waves.

It is clear that people, including children, can pretty quickly learn to do this. When they do, their brain-wave pattern does change. Nobody disputes that. The question is: what happens when they leave the office? (A related method uses passive brain-wave manipulation, feeding brain waves back into the brain via mild stimulation. The passive method is not much studied, so I focus here only on the active feedback methods.)

What Is the Claim? Two types of neurofeedback are commonly used. The first focus is on what is called the brain-wave spectrum—slow-wave versus fast-wave activity. Here the child learns to change the ratio of slow- to fast-wave activity (see Chapter 1 if you want to refresh yourself on how this is related to the idea of cortical arousal). The idea is attractive because, as reviewed in Chapter 1, many children with ADHD have excessive "slow wave" brain activity. In fact, this type of biofeedback has been proposed since the 1970s. However, in the last few years more sophisticated studies have attempted proper evaluation and better targeting of this method. The second method seeks to train slow cortical potentials, another particular kind of electrical brain signal, but the principle is the same.

In either case, the adjustment of brain electrical signals is thought to be associated with the best focus and alertness. The child views a feedback display while safe, painless electrodes on her head record her brain activity. The feedback display changes when the child is outside the desired zone. Again in the example we're using here, the display may show a ball or cartoon character on a screen, who will move into a certain area when the child achieves the targeted brain-wave pattern. Alternatively, the child views a movie, which stops if the child loses the brain-wave target. Feedback therefore continually tells the child how well she is hitting her brain wave target. In other words, this is a type of behavioral modification therapy, but it is modifying the child's mental arousal state. Usually the feedback is individually adjusted to help the child get enough positive feedback to avoid discouragement and stay engaged. Gradually, over several sessions, the idea is that the child learns to regulate her brain waves and, it is thought, to recognize when she is in a "calm-alert" state so she can bring herself into that state voluntarily and control her attention symptoms.

What Do the Data Show? Expert scientific reviews were published in 2013, 2014, and 2015. All painted the same picture. The most extensive (in 2014) concluded that these methods did not demonstrate the type of cortical learning that was intended. As with computerized training, behavioral and school effects were seen by raters who were least likely to be blind to the study and could have been influenced by their own expectations. When proper controls and blinded raters were looked at, effects tended to be small and unreliable.

Bottom Line. This treatment is not ready for prime time as an effective ADHD treatment, despite some fascinating progress and isolated promising results. Once again, serious science lies behind these ideas, and well-intentioned investigators are interested. However, once again, marketing and sales have outstripped R&D. These products are expensive, aggressively marketed, and easy to find, but unproven. Too often, the data shown for marketing purposes does not meet the strict standards of a well-controlled trial. The scientific consensus at this writing is that the passive method needs proper studies; meanwhile, the active learning method of neurofeedback is a potentially promising treatment, but not yet ready to recommend for your child. Stay tuned: future data may yet prove this stuff works. But for now, guard your wallet.

> At press time, science had not shown that biofeedback/neurofeedback was worth the investment for your child with ADHD.

DIRECT BRAIN STIMULATION

What Is It? The idea here is to directly stimulate the brain with a localized magnetic pulse or a gentle electrical current passed through the scalp. This is not old-fashioned electroconvulsive therapy (ECT), which is now given under anesthesia and uses a strong electric current to cause a brain seizure, attempting to "reset" the brain and flood it with positive neurotransmitters, and is used when other treatments aren't working. In contrast, the gentle current used in direct brain stimulation is given while awake and does not have any obvious behavioral or sensory impact at the moment it is given. Here I pull heavily from an authoritative review provided at the very end of 2015 in the *Journal of Child Neurology.*

What Are the Exact Methods? One method is called *transcranial magnetic stimulation* (TMS). It involves use of a coil placed near the head; an electrical current in the coil generates an electromagnetic pulse, which penetrates the skull and in turn alters electrical signaling in the brain.

The effect can be demonstrated. For example, if the pulse is directed at the motor cortex, motor signaling in the hand can be recorded by electrodes in the hand. If the pulse is directed at the visual cortex, the patient will report seeing a visual image. By varying the pulse frequency, the operator can cause inhibition or excitation of activity in the targeted brain region. This method has been proposed as a diagnostic tool, as a tool to improve medication effectiveness, and as a direct treatment for ADHD and other behavioral, mental, and emotional conditions. Although the method is generally seen as safe in adults, and is beginning to be evaluated for safety in children, some worrisome side effects can occur, including headaches and, very rarely, seizures. A consensus conference as early as 2009 suggested this tool was reasonably safe in children but that repetitive pulses should be used only with good clinical reason (for example, other treatments have failed).

A related method is *transcranial direct current stimulation* (TCS). Electrodes are placed on the scalp and an electrical current is passed through the scalp between the electrodes. While this method also can target a specific location, the effect is less targeted than for TMS. This method does not stimulate as much neural activity and so has less risk, but also may have less effectiveness due to being less focused.

These Sound Exciting. What Is the State of the Evidence? These truly are some of the most intriguing and potentially revolutionary treatments for psychiatric problems to emerge in many years. Some pilot findings are striking. As a result, the National Institute of Mental Health has invested heavily in research on these methods to see how far they can go. Both TMS and TCS have some evidence of benefit for depression, and possibly for other conditions like migraine. (Mechanisms like epigenetic change are unstudied.) There have been no proper controlled trials of TMS published in ADHD, although some are under way as of this writing. For TCS, a trial is under way for adults with ADHD as I write, but no results are yet available. I am aware of no trials in children with ADHD.

Bottom Line. For ADHD, these methods, while intriguing, are in the category of experimental, unproven treatments. Unfortunately, unscrupulous privateers may market them to you. Most important is that risks for children are not well described. For example, it is unknown whether stimulation that may improve one area (such as attention) may cause impairments in other areas (such as memory) in children. Until those risks are clarified and proper trials completed, avoid these methods for your child with ADHD.

> *TMS and TCS are intriguing new psychiatric treatments but are barely beginning to be studied. Avoid them for children until we learn much more about risks and benefits.*

 TAKE-HOME POINTS

Technology and ADHD

New high-tech computer-game-based and other methods of treating ADHD are fascinating and in some cases quite promising, but not yet ready for prime time. Keep an eye on these but don't spend money on them yet.

Computer and mobile screens and Internet are here to stay, and it's important to stay tuned in to your child's media and Internet use. Technological devices provide today's young people with social connection and unlimited information, but they also introduce unique risks for children with ADHD, particularly with regard to promoting aggression and opening the door to victimization. While the harmful effect of screen media on the development of attention appears to be slight, other risks are real and warrant following the steps in this chapter to keep your child with ADHD safe from the secondary harms that can occur.

6

Environmental Chemicals and ADHD

Sorting Alarm from Prudent Caution

Most of you have worried about chemical pollution and ADHD in relation to your child, while few of us know all the chemistry involved in what they do. Yet this difficult question is very important. It affects what products we buy, where we live, and how policymakers and businesspeople set their rules and regulations for commerce. Our watchword here will be vigilance without alarm: The risks are real and well documented in relation to ADHD, yet are sometimes sensationalized and at other times erroneously minimized by those who are not familiar with the latest findings. Some basic precautions can sharply contain those risks for your child. But to contain all the risks, policymakers will need to step up as well.

It was clear in recent public health crises around lead and other pollutants in 2015 and 2016 in the United States that many public officials, school officials, and others were not aware of the relevant science, either. That convinced me that it's important for you to know where we stand with ADHD and chemical pollution. Some solutions, unfortunately, will require action by policymakers. When we look to the future, it seems likely that this problem will get worse before it gets better, so staying ahead of the curve is our goal.

It makes sense that chemical pollution could affect the brain. After all, the brain's basic means of communication depends on chemicals—

neurotransmitters, hormones, trace metals, and other compounds. Thus, when chemicals enter the body from the outside, the nervous system tries to extract information from them. In the case of chemicals that were not present during evolutionary times and which our body does not expect (lead, synthetic plastics, chemical pesticides), or in the case of overdose of trace elements our body expects only at very scant doses (such as cadmium or arsenic), this "information" can and does disrupt the brain. (We've already discussed the chemical additives in food; see Chapter 3.)

As I am writing in 2016, chemical pollution is again in the headlines in relation to children's health. Here in Portland, Oregon, local glass factories were suspected of allowing harmful levels of cadmium and other chemicals into the air, while overall air quality is astonishingly poor for a prosperous, well-managed modern city, due to concentrations of diesel truck pollution through the heart of the city. But probably the biggest headlines of 2016 came from lead—maybe the oldest and most well-studied pollutant that affects children's brain development, and the most well established in its association with ADHD and other neurodevelopmental problems. The tragic release of leaded water into the community drinking supply in Flint, Michigan, and the subsequent discovery in community after community that lead levels in drinking water were unacceptable—all spoke to the challenge of putting an end to pollution once it has entered our environment. After all, lead was heavily regulated in the U.S. beginning over a generation ago. So, let's start with lead, in some detail, because it provides an excellent example of how research progresses and how toxicant pollution comes into our discussion. Then we'll examine other compounds in less detail, keeping the model of lead in mind to help us evaluate various claims both from science and from government and industry.

Lead

Lead is associated with ADHD, even at very low doses. This is confirmed in nationally representative surveys in the United States, Canada, and elsewhere, and its effects show up independent of numerous correlated variables. *It makes sense to take every precaution to limit or eliminate your child's exposure to lead.* This exposure can come from leaching of water pipes, air pollution from smokestacks, airplane exhaust, chipping paint in the home or school, or contaminated soil in areas where lead products were previously used. Leaded paint has also been found in some toys manufactured overseas.

So let's review the lead story. Authoritative background on toxicant exposures (and their interaction with micronutrients) was assembled more than a decade ago by the Association for Psychological Science's series *Psychological Science in the Public Interest*. I use it for some background but then draw on more recent work for current findings related to ADHD.

Lead, of course, naturally occurs on the earth. It is stable and inert, meaning it doesn't react or combine with other chemicals. As a result, the total amount on the earth does not change. During the evolutionary period, from 1 million years ago until 10,000 years ago, humans experienced very little exposure to lead. In fact, based on studies of bones of prehistoric humans, the average lead level in human blood during evolutionary times is speculated to have been about 0.16 parts per billion. We can tentatively think of this as the "normal" level of lead for humans.

Over the last 6,000 years, people mined and dug about 300 million tons of lead out of the ground and used it to make, in ancient times, pottery (particularly ill advised, as it turned out), weapons, agricultural tools, and mechanical parts and, in more recent times, numerous commercial and industrial products. Half of this has found its way back into a harmless location in the earth or in the ocean, but about 150 million tons are still in our human environment in some form. Due to air and water currents, they are widely dispersed to even the most remote areas of the earth.

> The average level of lead in the bodies of American and Canadian children and children in other nations is still 100 times the "normal" amount expected by evolution of our brain and body.

LEAD AND THE BRAIN: A HISTORY

Scientists can now describe in great detail how lead affects the brain. These effects in turn predict changes in behavior, attention, and IQ in children. Lead is fatal to children at ranges of 1,000 to 1,500 ppb (100 to 150 mcg/dL). During the nineteenth and twentieth centuries, the levels

FAQ: WHAT DOES "PARTS PER BILLION" SIGNIFY?

I know, I didn't say there would be math . . . but it's useful to have a grasp of what these measures of lead (and other contaminant) levels really mean, so here goes:

Lead is measured in micrograms per deciliter of blood (mcg/dL). A microgram is one billionth of a kilogram. A deciliter is one tenth of a liter. In blood, a gram is about equal to a milliliter (1 kilogram = 1 liter in water; blood and water have similar densities). A milliliter is one thousandth of a liter. So a gram is one thousandth of a liter or one hundredth of a deciliter. A microgram therefore is one millionth of a gram or one billionth of a liter, or one hundred-millionth of a deciliter. Thus, 1 microgram per deciliter is 1 part per 100 million. Multiplying this by 10, 1 mcg/dL is 10 parts per billion (ppb). The scientific literature uses mcg/dL, but to make it easier to follow I've converted to ppb. The evolutionary amount of lead was calculated from ancient skeletons and converted to an estimated blood level of 0.016 mcg/dL, which I then multiply by 10 to arrive at 0.16 ppb. If we multiply this by 100 we get 16 parts per 100 billion or about 1 part per 10 billion. When lead is measured in the blood, we see in children on average 1 mcg/dL (10 mcg/l or 10 ppb)—that is, about 100 times the projected "normal" level in evolutionary times. And this is after regulating lead in gasoline and paint.

among American children spiked to around 300 ppb *on average*, with thousands of children killed and many others sickened and permanently injured by lead poisoning. This was the direct result of unrestrained commercial and industrial use of lead in gasoline, house paint, water pipes, and other commercial products during that era. To the shame of some industries and politicians, restricting it was vigorously resisted despite the evidence of harm.

Lead use was finally restricted from the 1970s to the 1990s in the United States, Canada, and Europe, and was then phased out of gasoline and paint. By the 2000s, the average lead level among children in the United States had dropped dramatically, from about 200 ppb in the 1970s to 10 ppb. This average masks wide variation. Low-income and racial and ethnic minority children can have average levels that are much higher; and children in other nations that do not regulate lead still have levels far higher than those in the United States.

It's important for those of you getting clinical testing for your child to realize that clinical testing in many locales is often not as sensitive as the tests we do in our research. In our studies, we can detect lead in 99 percent of the children we test—but we test with a sensitivity down to 0.3 mcg/dL or 3 ppb. Many clinical tests have only one-tenth of that sensitivity, reaching only about 3 mcg/dL or 30 ppb, so that nearly every child would test as "zero lead" or "no detectable lead." Technicians will tell you your child's level is "zero" or "safe" because it is undetectable. That is the conventional position. Is it good enough? No.

"SAFE" LEAD LEVEL AND ADHD

When levels were very high in the twentieth century, lead's association with ADHD and lower IQ was very clear in the literature. Controversy over the lead level that actually caused ADHD and lower IQ arose from 1990 to 2010 as lead levels in the population dropped: was there still

---

FAQ: HOW CAN WE BE SURE LEAD TESTS OF OUR CHILD ARE ACCURATE?

You can ask what the minimum detectable threshold was in the test your child received. If it was able to detect down to under 1 mcg/dL, then you should be fine with a negative or "clean" test. But if you find out the minimum detectable threshold was 2 or 3 mcg/dL, and you're worried about your child's attention or intellectual development, or you have reason to be concerned about lead in the child's environment, advocate for a repeat using a more sensitive method such as inductively coupled plasma mass spectrometry (ICP-MS). This method is expensive and therefore not used in routine testing in many places because special labs have to be used. But it is available. Also don't rely on a finger prick; a regular blood draw from the arm vein is more accurate.

> Many standard clinical lead-level tests detect only down to 30 parts per billion, so a child with a lead level under that amount will be pronounced as having "no detectable lead" but in fact may still have a high enough lead level to affect brain development.

an association between these lower levels and neurodevelopmental problems? However, in the 2000s a series of studies, including representative national population surveys as well as studies by our group that used a case control method (taking children with carefully evaluated ADHD and comparing to children without ADHD), all showed the effects on ADHD remained. Even when average lead levels were as low as 10 ppb (1 mcg/dL, the national average at that time), slight variations in lead (from, say, 6 to 12 ppb or 0.6 to 1.2 mcg/dL in blood) were still associated with reduced IQ and increased chances of having ADHD. This confirmed that *if there is a "safe" level of lead for children, it is below the detection limit of even our most advanced mass spectroscopy instruments.* Animal studies looking at lower doses also saw effects. Thus, we had most of the pieces of the puzzle, and national authorities lowered the official "safe" level of lead in the 2000s for the third time, to 50 ppb (5 mcg/dL); but probably the "safe" level is really only a small fraction of that. At these lower levels, however, it seems likely that lead has minimal effect on many children and now is affecting a vulnerable subset to a greater extent than the others. Let me explain.

Could Lead Really Be Causal in ADHD? Aren't There a Lot of Other Explanations? This is the key question. The correlations are worrisome, and animal studies use random assignment to show that lead causes hyperactivity in rats or mice. But human behavior seems more complex—humans live in uncontrolled environments, so an unimaginable list of possible alternative explanations, what scientists call "unmeasured confounds," could explain a correlation of lead level with ADHD. For example, maybe kids with higher lead also have worse diets or more stress; the list of possibilities is almost endless. To see if the effect is causal, we used a method called "genomic stratification." This is a "natural experiment" where nature's random assignment of genes helps us. Lead in the body is a metal—it interacts with other metals, particularly iron. (Iron, of course, is a nutrient, but lead is not.) Because the body depends on iron, we have genes that take charge of how iron is handled, how it is metabolized and excreted. Well, when they run into lead, these genes start to affect lead as well—either directly or indirectly, due to lead's interaction with iron.

The version of these genes you have influences how fast or efficiently your body handles iron and thus how your body handles lead. The different forms of these genes (called mutations) are assigned, by nature, to the population at random. We therefore have a natural experiment in which people are randomly assigned to high and low efficiency of metabolizing lead and iron. If the association of lead with ADHD is affected by this random genetic assignment, a causal effect is hard to deny.

And that's just what we saw when we studied this (the result was published in 2016 in *Psychological Science*). The association of lead with ADHD, even at levels of only 10 ppb, was much stronger depending on which iron metabolism gene a child had. This also illustrates that for some children, the association of lead with ADHD at levels around 1 ppb is minimal; but for other children, depending on their genetic makeup, that association remains substantial.

Lead and Epigenetics. Lead's effect on the brain may well be epigenetic—that is, due to chemical changes in DNA in the brain that create a stable change in gene expression and change brain function and behavior. Several studies have asked that question. In a study published in 2014, researchers at Hefei Technology University in China gave rats lead in their drinking water and randomly assigned them to no lead, low levels (intended to be similar to the typical human population level currently), and high levels (like the population level in past decades). They measured the animals' "hyperactivity" by looking at excess movement in exploring a new room. The "normal" rats showed efficient exploration of the room with little wasted activity. The "low-dose" rats showed excessive and inefficient exploration, suggesting "hyperactivity." The "high-dose" rats also had excess activity, but not as much as the low-dose rats, suggesting they were overactive but also sick from the lead. Both of the groups that were exposed to lead showed changes in their brain chemistry, and their brain tissue was later subjected to analysis to see if there were epigenetic changes. In this case, they looked at a type of epigenetic change called *histone modifications*. In fact, the team observed such changes notably in the hippocampus, a brain area important for learning and self-regulation. The effects were still present after the animals died, so while we don't

The effects of higher-than-normal lead levels in the blood are a classic example of how an epigenetic change in the brain influences ADHD.

know if they were permanent, they were sustained for a period of time. A statistical analysis suggested that these changes could statistically account for the behavior changes caused by the lead dosing.

Caveats: What We Still Don't Know. We don't know:

- If at some very low level lead is harmless.

- When in development its damage is done (are there critical periods?). However, postnatal exposure appears to be at least as important as prenatal exposure in the case of lead (this is not true of all chemicals).

- Whether the key factor is total cumulative exposure or peak exposure amount.

The bottom line: The weight of evidence suggests that lead, even at levels typical in American children today (remember, still possibly 100 times the likely normal level during evolution), contributes to ADHD and that it is plausible that it does so through epigenetic changes affecting the brain. As research has progressed, scientists have learned that levels once thought to be safe, and seemingly tiny, are still

---

 FOR DETAILS ON THE SCIENCE . . .

If you're interested in reading the details of the article in *Psychological Science in the Public Interest,* it is available in the publication's online archive:

Neurotoxicants, micronutrients, and social environments: Individuals and combined effects on children's development (December 2005), vol. 6, no. 3. Available online at *www.psychologicalscience.org/index.php/publications/journals/pspi/pspi-archive.*

If you're interested in reading about the rat study that showed how lead exposure caused an epigenetic change that in turn caused symptoms resembling ADHD, look up:

Luo, M., Xu, Y., Cai, R., Tang, Y., Ge, M. M., Liu, Z. H., et al. (2014). Epigenetic histone modification regulates developmental lead exposure induced hyperactivity in rats. *Toxicology Letters, 225*(1), 78–85.

harmful during early development. Lead is a good illustration of the general problems with environmental toxicants and their possible relation to ADHD.

Other Chemicals

If lead were the only chemical we had to worry about, we might be okay. The point that bothers parents is that there are too many chemicals to keep track of. This is a fair complaint. The chemical revolution of the twentieth century has resulted in an explosion of chemical products that have entered children's environments. Over 80,000 chemicals are in commercial use. The *neurotoxic profile* (that is, how much they interfere with children's brain functioning) is unknown for nearly all of these. Fewer than 1,000 of these chemicals have well-characterized neurotoxic profiles, and even in those, the effects on small children are often poorly studied. However, some are very well studied, have known neurotoxic effects, even at low doses, and are common in the environment so that most children have some exposure. They represent a major policy headache for political leaders, a major challenge for business, and a significant worry for parents. Advocacy groups have sounded alarm bells and tried to get better regulation. After years of inaction, in 2016 the U.S. Congress updated a thirty-year-old law to try to improve regulation of chemicals in consumer products and commercial use, to the partial relief of many advocates but still probably with insufficient protections overall.

What other chemicals are of most concern? Public news outlets have given considerable coverage in recent

> Of the 80,000 chemicals in commercial use today, we have a good understanding of how much they interfere with children's brain functioning for fewer than 1,000.

years to plastics such as BPA (bisphenol A), a synthetic that can leach out of consumer products into the human body. Concern has continued for decades about ongoing air pollution from smokestack sources that expose us to mercury and cadmium, as well as lead and other compounds—the damaging health effects on children and adults of mercury in air and water pollution are well established. But there is also growing concern about pollutants from vehicles such as fine particulate matter, nitrogen oxides, and polycyclic aromatic hydrocarbons.*

Unfortunately, it's very difficult to keep your children from exposure to potentially neurotoxic chemicals. They get toxic chemicals into their bodies by mouthing toys and other objects; eating food with pesticides; drinking water with toxins in it; breathing air pollution; and absorbing chemicals through their skin. The primary route depends on the particular pollutant involved. At the same time, the effect of these chemicals on children's development is notoriously difficult to study, because we obviously can't do a gold standard random-assignment experiment like we can with diet or exercise. The question parents most ask me is, with such a complicated picture, "How worried should I be?" and in particular, "What can I do?" We want to avoid alarm but maintain prudence, and we'll try to strike a balance here by hitting the highlights of what we know and a few basic recommendations for protecting your child with ADHD.

A list of the major classes of chemicals of concern is in the box on the next page.

The level of evidence available for the different classes of chemicals varies, but for several of them we have all the evidence needed to draw conclusions.

ORGANIC POLLUTANTS AND ENDOCRINE-DISRUPTING CHEMICALS

Many of these chemicals are called *persistent organic pollutants* because they remain in the body for a long time and comprise organic molecules such as carbon. Many are referred to as "endocrine disrupters" because they can exert effects by mimicking hormone action in the body. For example, some chemicals occupy estrogen receptors. In animals, these chemicals can fool the body into changing sexual development and cre-

---

*A recent review concluded these emissions from gasoline and diesel vehicles are likely related to autism risk and lower IQ, but that evidence related to ADHD is still inconclusive and no causal studies have been conducted in humans. One large population study showed a risk for ADHD but another large study did not. See Suades-Gonzalez, E., Gascon, M., Guxens, M., & Sunye, J. (2016). Air pollution and neuropsychological development: A review of latest evidence. *Endocrinology, 156*, 3473–3482.

EXAMPLES OF KNOWN NEUROTOXIC CHEMICALS IN COMMON USE

Pollutant	Association with child developmental problems
Metals	
Lead	Definite
Mercury	Definite
Cadmium	Likely
Manganese	Suspected
Organic pollutants	
BHP	Suspected
BPA	Likely
PCBs	Definite
PBBs	Likely
Organophosphate pesticides	Likely

ating downstream effects on brain neurotransmission patterns. That has led to concern that these types of chemicals may cause early puberty or other effects in children, as well as affecting cognitive development.

When chemicals are known to be harmful to the brain, they are called *neurotoxicants*. Some, like some pesticides, are neurotoxic by design. Others are neurotoxic incidentally, which is discovered by research. Many of the chemicals of concern today are known neurotoxicants.

Persistent organic pollutants include chemicals that have received extensive publicity in the past, like PCBs (polychlorinated biphenyls), as well as related chemicals that have received more recent publicity, such as BPA (bisphenol A) and phthalates. Naturally, scientists have had more time to investigate chemicals that have been in use longer and less time to study chemicals introduced more recently. So our information is more definitive for chemicals that have been around longer—and often are now being phased out due to the results of this independent research. The box on page 149 lists several classes of these chemicals and conveys some of the dizzying array of plastic-type and endocrine-disrupting types of chemicals. These have myriad uses, including in industry, electronics, and manufacturing, but also in many household products. Typically, at least some of them can be found in household dust, food, water, and household products including toys, shampoos, and food containers.

ORGANIC NEUROTOXICANT CHEMICALS

Class of chemical	Chemicals	Sample sources
Perfluorinated alkyl acids	PFOS, PFOA	Teflon, water repellants, food, dust
Organochlorine pesticides	HCB, DDE, DDT	Agricultural use (phasing out)
Organophosphate pesticides	DAP, chlorpyrifos	Food (agricultural), household
Nondioxin-like PCBs	PCB-153	Industrial sites; fatty food
Brominated flame retardants	PBDE-47, PBDE-99	Furniture, bedding, mattresses
Phthalates	DBP	Plastic toys, plastic dishes
Organohalogens (OHCs)	4OH-CB-146	Adhesives, plastics, electronics
Others	BPA, PCE	Plastics, food containers, shampoo

Key: PFOS, perfluorooctane sulfonate; PFOA, perfluorooctanoic acid; HCB, hexachlorobenzene; DDE, dichlorodiphenyldichloroethylene; DDT, dichlorodiphenyltrichloroethane; DAP, dialkyl phosphate; PCB, polychlorinated biphenyl; PBDE, polybrominated diphenyl ether; DBP, dibutyl phthalate; OH-CB, hydroxylated polychlorinated biphenyls; BPA, bisphenol A; PCE, perchloroethylene or tetrachloroethylene.

Note: Data based in part on de Cock, M., Maas, Y.G., & van de Bor, M. (2012). Does perinatal exposure to endocrine disruptors induce autism spectrum and attention deficit hyperactivity disorders? Acta Paediatrica, 101, 811–818.

Exposure is nearly universal around the world because these chemicals are stored in body fat and then transmitted up the food chain. Nearly everyone in the world has detectable levels of these chemicals in their body tissues (such as urine, blood, or breast milk). In 2015, the Endocrine Society's second annual consensus scientific statement noted substantial data linking this class of chemicals to obesity and diabetes, female reproduction, male reproduction, hormone-sensitive cancers in females, prostate cancer, thyroid, and the neurodevelopmental and neuroendocrine systems—that is, brain health. Sex-specific effects may be relevant because the brain early on develops differently in girls and boys due to prenatal variation in testosterone. As a result, boys and girls may have different behavior responses to these early, widespread exposures. One small survey study supported that supposition. However, when it comes to ADHD and neurodevelopment, sex-specific effects remain unclear in humans, so I do not emphasize them. These hormonally active chemicals may also disrupt development at puberty—a possibility beginning to be studied in animals but also having too little conclusive data for me to emphasize. That said, the early neurodevelopmental piece is my focus here. I will walk through just a couple of these key chemicals and major findings to give a sense of what we know about their role in problems like ADHD. I'll start with an older set of these chemicals because they are very well studied and can give us a picture of what we are likely to discover with newer but very similar chemicals going forward.

Organic Pollutants and Epigenetics. A major scientific review in 2015 summarized the literature on epigenetic findings and organic pollutants. While only a few specific chemicals have been studied, the results are clear. These pollutants exert epigenetic effects in development, which can be carried over to future generations (that is, can be inherited). These include pesticides as well as the other organic pollutants and plastics like BPA, of which the most well studied is an older chemical called PCBs (discussed next).

Once again, we have to wonder about causality. We have to rely heavily on animal studies because we cannot randomly assign people to chemical exposure. But here, too, different types of studies, like the following, keep pointing in the same direction for some of these organic pollutants:

- Prospective human studies (following forward to see if exposure variation predicts future outcome)

- Clinical studies (showing higher amounts of the chemicals in kids with neurodevelopmental disorders)

- Random assignment in animal studies showing causal effects on brain and behavior

- Mendelian randomization studies (parallel to our study of lead described earlier in this chapter) also supporting a causal role of organic pollutants in neurodevelopmental delays

For example, I'll mention one relatively recent study looking at this in rodents. Pregnant animals were exposed to vinclozolin, a fungicide commonly used on vegetables and fruits. It is an endocrine disruptor that can block the action of testosterone as well as alter estrogen and progesterone effects in development. It is being phased out now due to numerous studies of its risks. In this study, animals were randomly assigned to this exposure in a controlled experiment so that causality could be studied. The offspring had numerous epigenetic changes caused by the exposure, seen in their brains. The "grandchildren" also showed these effects, even though they had zero exposure. Thus, these organic pollutants can sometimes cause epigenetic changes in the brain that can persist across generations. This could be one source of their effects on development. Let's look further at the effects of this class of chemicals.

> Pesticide exposure can cause damage to future generations, not just the generation exposed to the chemicals.

PCBs. The most well-studied group of persistent organic pollutants is called PCBs. These were widely used industrial compounds (there are over a hundred in the PCB family and in a related group called PBBs or polybrominated biphenyls, as well as polybrominated diphenyl ethers, or PBDEs). They are chemical cousins of newer, less well-studied organic compounds like BPA that have replaced them.

PCBs were banned in the United States a generation ago due to all the studies showing, after years of their commercial use, that they harm humans. But like lead, they remain in the food chain for a long time. Thus, while their levels in human tissue are declining, they are not yet gone. Findings on PCBs are quite instructive because their chemical action is similar to that in many newer products still in use, including BPA and others, for which evidence is starting to emerge but is not yet as developed.

PCBs and related chemicals have become widely dispersed around the world and have been found at low levels in the body tissues of essentially all populations sampled, from the Inuit in the far north to the mainland American population and others around the world. Although in most people the amount of exposure is "low," just like with lead, this doesn't make it safe. Levels of 1–10 ppb are similar to levels that the body looks for when responding to its natural chemical messengers like hormones. A review in the 1990s concluded that the average population level was 2–10 ppb, enough to have an effect in the body's chemical signaling systems. Those levels in the population are steadily dropping now that manufacture of PCBs has been banned, but levels are no doubt increasing for other, related chemicals that have entered the mainstream in the meantime. Many of these other chemicals also show troubling associations, as noted below. And similar effects may occur with still other unstudied chemicals that are chemically related to PCBs, which also are meanwhile *increasing*. So let's look at what was learned about PCBs and see if it might prove to be true also of newer chemicals like BPA.

The current levels of organic chemicals in many people's bodies are similar to the natural levels of our own hormones experienced by the body during development. A series of landmark studies was done by Susan Rice and colleagues twenty years ago in monkeys. They dosed the monkeys with levels of PCB exposure that were similar to what the typical human exposure was in the United States at that time (in the 1990s). They found that on laboratory tasks that required development of prefrontal cortex, such as working memory, PCBs caused developmental problems. A crucial detail: the problems did not emerge until the young monkeys had started to mature, when their prefrontal cortex came "online" to handle the challenging cognitive problems the experimenters were giving them. When the monkeys were younger, they did not yet show deficits because none of the monkeys, in early life, had engaged that part of their brain that handles hard memory problems. Because this finding was parallel to the problems seen in ADHD, those authors argued by analogy that PCBs could contribute to ADHD. A number of human studies at that time added to the picture, finding that early-life PCB level predicted the later amount of problems with attention or cognitive development.

It is important to realize that these studies are difficult to design. Some chemicals work the opposite of others, making the interactions difficult to evaluate. Dispute has gone on as to the relative importance of prenatal versus postnatal exposure. In monkeys and rats, mothers exposed to PCBs behave differently with their offspring, further complicating the picture as to what causes what.

However, the known biological action of these chemicals, the human prospective studies, and the animal experiments converge to a reasonable probability that these types of chemicals play a role in disrupting the normal development of prefrontal cortex functioning and of advanced attention.

All is not lost, however. There's a lot we may be able to do to protect our children (and ourselves) even if we can't always (or immediately) eliminate toxic pollutants from our environment. For example, at least two studies have suggested that breastfeeding exerts a protective effect. These are obviously correlational studies because we cannot randomly assign chemical pollution in a human experiment. But these studies measured umbilical cord blood levels of organic pollutants when babies were born. They then kept track of their cognitive and behavioral development. Level of cord blood chemicals predicted infant development—but the effect disappeared among children whose mothers breastfed for an extended period. While we don't know if the effect was caused by the breastfeeding experience, something in breast milk, or other correlated factors (maybe these mothers were healthier or had better relationships with their babies), the results indicate that the chemical effects on development can be reversed. The box on the next page lists some other discoveries about possible protective effects against chemical exposures.

BPA (bisphenol A). BPA is a family of plastic compounds found in numerous consumer products, from children's toys to plastic utensils and food containers to shampoos. Unfortunately, laboratory studies have reported that they can leach out of these products during use. This is

LIFESTYLE FACTORS THAT MAY REDUCE THE DAMAGE DONE BY POLLUTANTS

Of course two children can be exposed to the same amounts and types of pollutants and not suffer the same damage. As noted earlier in this chapter, humans live in uncontrolled (versus lab) conditions, and many factors interact to affect their health. This knowledge gives us the power to apply some "antidotes" for pollutant exposure.

For example, both diet and stress appear to modify pollutant effects on children, giving us clues about how to protect them. Two studies in humans found that breastfeeding erased the effect of PCB exposure during gestation. This raises the possibility that sufficiently good early caregiving and nutrition can protect children's brain development and attention from at least some of these pollution effects. Having sufficient dietary iron may protect to some degree against lead exposure.

Other research has shown that pollutant effects on the brain are magnified when animals are stressed, suggesting another route to reduce effects by managing stress (perhaps via exercise or mindfulness; see Chapter 7). These offsetting effects, seen in animals, are still a bit speculative in humans—but this may be where the hockey puck ends up.

an obvious risk if young children chew on these items. However, maternal exposure during pregnancy (via food containers, hygiene products, and other sources) is an equal concern as chemicals leach off during use and can cross the placental barrier. Over 90 percent of the population has measurable levels of BPA in their bodies, suggesting that exposure is nearly universal. Because BPA affects sex hormones (such as steroid receptors in the brain), it affects the brain's sexually related development. Once again, some studies suggest that effects on behavior are different for boys and girls. There is clearer evidence for effects on children's emotional difficulties (anxiety, depression) than on ADHD, but also some evidence of effects on attention and aggression. There is also a tendency across studies for effects on childhood behavior problems to be clearer in slightly older children (age five) than in infants. This may be related to the earlier monkey findings of "sleeper" effects that emerge with maturation of the frontal cortex as it comes "online," as we saw in Rice's studies of PCBs.

Animal studies have suggested that early-life exposure (prenatally, most often) can interfere with brain development, cognition, and behavior in offspring and that there may be epigenetic mechanisms. The major human studies are the following:

- A study of several hundred women in Cincinnati reported that prenatal BPA levels in the mother predicted poor executive functioning and more hyperactivity in girls but not in boys by age three to four years.

- A similar cohort study in California followed children to nine years of age (to date) and reported increases in anxiety, depression, and behavior problems in boys for prenatal exposure, and in girls for childhood exposures.

- A study of 193 pregnant women in New York found that their prenatal BPA levels predicted their offspring's behavior problems, particularly emotional reactivity, but only in boys and only for prenatal (not subsequent childhood) exposures.

- A recent review of all the human studies in this area found only those listed above and a few others. But the effects were consistent in showing that early-life (usually prenatal) exposure levels were associated with offspring behavior problems, including inattention.

- As proof that the exposures are coming from everyday products (and that you can do something about it), a recent study taught teenage girls to monitor the ingredients in their personal care products (shampoo, soap, makeup). The recorded chemical levels in their bodies subsequently dropped by over 30 percent in a short period of time.

The bottom line: The picture for BPA is starting to be very reminiscent of the picture for PCBs.

Phthalates. Phthalates are colorless, odorless liquids. They are called plasticizers or softeners. For example, they soften PVC (polyvinyl chloride) products like food packages, tubing, and toys, and personal care products like nail polish. They are also used in vinyl flooring and wall covering. They easily escape from the product into the air in the house or car (that "new car" smell). Again, exposure is widespread; 75–90 percent of the U.S. population had measurable levels in their body in one national survey conducted by the national Centers for Disease Control and Prevention (CDC) about a decade ago—use of this class of chemical has since increased.

Phthalates became infamous because they leach into food that is heated in plastic containers, hence the common warning not to put plastic containers in the microwave. They can also leach out of plastic toys when children chew on them. At least three of the phthalates have been banned from consumer products, cosmetics, and toys in the United States as evidence from independent studies of their damaging effects has mounted, but others are still in use, as they have not yet been studied enough to be banned. The chemicals are, unfortunately for our children, "innocent until proven guilty" and like lead was in the past, they are well defended by their industry sponsors. But we can predict where the story will go for most of this class of chemicals—they are probably harmful to children's brain development.

The boxes—the types of studies needed to decide whether they are related to ADHD or to brain development—have been starting to get checked off just in the last five years. The results, once again, are concerning. Again, we look for different kinds of data. A case control study of nearly 200 children and a nationally representative survey of nearly 1,500 children each showed that phthalate level in the child's body was associated with ADHD. In the national survey, the average level of individual phthalates (metabolites in urine) in children was 5–50 ppb; the accumulated total of all the chemicals looked at was about 100 ppb. Age, sex, race, living in poverty, co-occurring lead level, or maternal smoking all failed to explain the association. Possibly due to their action via sex hormones, phthalate effects were larger in girls in some studies.

Prenatal levels in urine of pregnant women were also associated with offspring problems with inattention, impulsivity, and hyperactivity. At least two animal experiments showed that phthalate exposure *caused* hyperactivity in rats, and at least three animal studies showed that exposure causally disrupted brain development. In humans, the case control study of nearly 200 children (done in Korea) found phthalate levels were associated with reduced brain development in key brain regions observed in MRI brain imaging. Levels in the children were about 50 ppb in that study.

The bottom line: While we don't yet have causal studies in humans, the research boxes checked off so far are consistent with early-life phthalate exposure contributing to ADHD, parallel to the story seen in the past for lead, PCBs, and other chemicals.

Pesticides. A final area I'll mention is pesticides because this one is fairly easy for you to address. These are relevant because they are also everywhere—sprayed around schools to control weeds, on food crops, and in household pest sprays. Older pesticides had the bad quality of persisting on food for a long time, so there was a real issue of eating pesticides in our fruits and vegetables from the supermarket. In some instances, these were very difficult to wash off. The current type of crop pesticide (called *organophosphate pesticides*) dissolves more quickly in water and in sunlight and so is intended to be safer for consumers (although the immediate effects are more severe, so it poses equal or greater risks for farmworkers who are exposed). But as with other pollutants, regulatory agencies have tended to look at gross health effects in adult animals and neglected careful study of the subtle effects of low-level exposure on the developing brain in children—particularly the ever-sensitive prefrontal cortex in nonhuman primates and humans. In that vein, it is notable that one particular study showed that children eating only organic fruits and vegetables had negligible urine levels of any organophosphate pesticide compared to children eating a "standard" diet of fruits and vegetables.

> To keep a constructive perspective on what you can do about pollutants, remember that many factors affect whether a potential toxin harms an individual. We can take hope in controlling what **is** in our control.

The bottom line: While data are not yet definitive, chemical pesticides are a possible risk for your child's brain that are relatively easily avoided.

Stress Increases the Harm Done by Pollutants

We've already discussed how diet and pollutants interact in development, with one amplifying or protecting against the other. I also briefly mentioned stress, but it's important to note that the definition of *stress* really applies here. *More and more research suggests that the effects of poor diet, and the effects of pollution or toxicants, are amplified by emotional or psychological stress.* This is particularly important in relation to psychological stress experienced by the mother during pregnancy. But it probably also applies to stress experienced by the young child. Chapter 7 talks about managing stress.

This makes sense when we think about it. All of these factors (poor diet, pollution, psychological stress) are a stress on the child's body. The mind and body cannot be separated. The brain and the body work as a single whole. All the body and brain recognize is incoming stress, which can combine to overload their ability to cope biologically. As briefly noted in Chapter 2, these different stressors may share many biological pathways, so they can counteract and interact with one another. The next chapter goes into detail about how psychological stress and ADHD interact.

 TAKE-HOME POINTS

Environmental Chemicals

In light of the fact that any stressor is going to increase the damage done by pollutants, the best way to look at your child's exposure to chemicals is to try to reduce whatever you can control in this overall "matrix of risk." That way, you can worry less about the things you can't control. I may not know about all the air pollution in my neighborhood, for example, but I can make sure we eat healthy food and keep our family's stress level manageable.

Many public officials still undersell the risks of chemical pollution to children in relation to ADHD and neural development generally. In part this is intended to avoid causing alarm, and in part it is a holdover from the past when it was assumed—wrongly—that if a child was not physically sick, he was not being hurt. Now we know that it's little consolation to find that adult animals don't get cancer when exposed to a certain dose of chemical. Fractions of the cancer-causing dosage are enough to disrupt brain function and development in human children. We saw that ADHD is related even to levels of lead previously considered safe and probably to several organic pollutants as well. At these lower levels it's likely that some kids are not much affected while others are quite sensitive, based on their genetic makeup as well as other factors like stress. These genotype × environment interactions are not yet mapped well enough to enable us to test your child for sensitivity to these chemicals. Thus, prudence suggests minimizing your child's exposure to help combat ADHD (and prevent it).

> *The fact that some children are affected by even so-called low-level or everyday chemical exposure is likely due in part to their genetic makeup. In the future we may be able to map these gene x environment interactions to help further protect those at risk.*

 AT A GLANCE

Action Steps to Reduce the Harm of Exposure to Chemical Pollutants

As I said at the beginning of this chapter, your mantra here should be "vigilance without alarm." Human children's brains are even more "plastic" or responsive to their environment than the brains of other animals. It's why human kids can learn almost anything—for good or for ill. Because of this, it makes sense to take precautions. On the other hand, alarm about chemical risks can simply lead to bewilderment and a sense of helplessness—and many children likely will have no noticeable consequences from everyday exposures. The prudent steps to reduce chemical exposure and its possible effects on your child are:

1. Urge policymakers to further strengthen requirements for product safety in relation to new and existing chemicals on the market to which children are exposed.

2. Be vigilant about possible chemical exposures and take the precautions you can, including:

   - Don't assume a product is safe just because it is legal. Notice ingredients. Encourage your kids to track the toxic chemical ingredients in their personal care products and consider alternatives. At least one study shows this can reduce their exposure to organic pollutants by 30 percent or more.

- If you are pregnant and can do so, breastfeed for at least twelve months after birth.

- If your home was built before 1980, dust frequently and immediately repair any chipped or peeling paint. The U.S. Environmental Protection Agency provides a thorough summary of how to protect your home from lead at *www.epa.gov/lead/protect-your-family-exposures-lead*.

- Consider a reverse osmosis or other high-quality water filter for drinking water. Select a filter certified for lead by NSF (*http://info.nsf.org/Certified/DWTU*), the Water Quality Association (*www.wqa.org*), or Underwriters Laboratories (*www.ul.com*).

- Remove chemical pesticides/herbicides from your home and use extremely rarely if ever. Research safe cleaning alternatives.

- Tolerate weeds in the yard or weed by hand.

- Fight pests with nontoxic methods:
    - Use integrated pest management methods to make your home inhospitable to pests (get started at the EPA website).
    - Use nontoxic options like boric acid to kill or deter pests when needed.
    - The Northwest Center for Alternatives to Pesticides provides pest-specific ideas at *www.pesticide.org/resources_for_pests*.

- Purchase organic produce to minimize chemical pesticides on your food (see Chapter 3).

- Feed your children a healthy diet that can help protect against chemical pollution, including sufficient iron, zinc, protein, and omega-3 fatty acids (see Chapter 3).

- Be mindful of potential leaching of chemicals from plastic toys that children may chew on. Washington and Oregon have websites listing products marketed for children that contain potentially toxic chemicals.

- Manage stress—see Chapter 7.

7

Adversity, Stress, Trauma, and ADHD

Finding Sanctuary

If I asked you to check off from a list of adjectives ten that describe your life and your child's, chances are you would check "stressful." Many experts think life is getting more stressful for most people, for many reasons. ADHD in a child multiplies parental stress as well as child stress. Further, the child with ADHD is less stress-resilient than other kids, as noted in Chapter 1 and described below.

When Keisha came to me for consultation, she was already unhappy with her son's doctor. "His doctor says he has ADHD. That doesn't make any sense! Look at what we are dealing with. We live in a poor neighborhood; there's gang violence all the time; in the winter our heat was shut off because I couldn't pay the bills and we were freezing. And I've got three kids sharing a tiny bedroom! What about all that?"

Keisha makes a good point. Sufficient trauma or adversity can cause a child to look just like he has ADHD. The official diagnostic system doesn't treat this any differently from ADHD in a better environment— but the label can feel pretty inadequate if you are facing lots of adversity. And if there is sufficient emotional trauma, the resulting problems with self-regulation really need to be understood as something other than ADHD—in fact, they require a different therapeutic approach than is usually applied for ADHD.

Despite all this, historically stress and adversity are something of a "blind spot" in books about ADHD and maybe as a result, among doctors, clinicians, and counselors evaluating and treating ADHD. This is ironic and unfortunate for several reasons in light of recent science. First, as I'll outline in this chapter, *adversity can increase the chances of ADHD*. Second, *kids with ADHD seem to experience more adversity and serious stress than other kids*—both by bad luck and as a consequence of their own difficulties in self-regulation. Third, *kids with ADHD seem to be more sensitive to the effects of adversity when it occurs*—they are more likely to show the worst effects of adversity.

Thus, the problem really multiplies for kids with ADHD, magnifying the importance of trying to prevent or remedy risky experiences as well as taking a look at stress in the home and, to the extent you can, elsewhere in your child's life. We'll talk about how to do that here. In other chapters, we also look at specific kinds of risks to which kids with ADHD are susceptible, such as violent media and the unique risks of the Internet (Chapter 5). On the upside, the sensitivity to events of children with ADHD may turn out to represent sensitivity to the world in all respects, not just to adversity but also to healthy opportunity— a point explored below.

One of the most dramatic discoveries in the past decade has been a detailed understanding of the biological effects of chronic psychological stress on child development. It turns out these effects dovetail with interference in the biology and behavior of self-regulation. The effects can be far-reaching and can be seen physiologically (such as in heart rate response), hormonally (blood, saliva, and urine hormone secretion), in brain development (both in MRI imaging of children and in laboratory animals whose brains were later examined under a microscope), and in epigenetic and developmental changes both in people and in animals. Since kids with ADHD are often exposed to

> *The triple whammy of stress for kids vulnerable to ADHD:*
>
> 1. *Adversity can increase the risk of ADHD.*
>
> 2. *Children with ADHD seem to experience more stress and adversity than others even after taking into account potential stress inputs to ADHD.*
>
> 3. *Kids with ADHD seem to be more sensitive to the adversity they do experience.*

more chronic stress than others, and are probably more sensitive to it, the relevance of stress to their development moves to center stage.

How Stress and Adversity Can Increase the Risk of Self-Regulation Problems and ADHD

In other chapters we talk about biological stressors like poor diet (Chapter 3) and toxic chemicals (Chapter 6). In this chapter, I'm focusing on the more usual meaning of stress, that is, social or emotional stress and adversity. Adversity just means sustained or repeated hardship that provokes ongoing and substantial stress. That is intended to distinguish it from the routine stress of daily hassles.

Most of what we know about effects of stress comes either from studies of animals subjected to the equivalent of quite substantial stress on repeated occasions, or from human studies involving stressful events such as job loss, violence, or emotional abuse. In that sense we know more about adversity than about the cumulative effects of routine daily hassles that wear kids and parents out. We'll unpack the idea of adversity more in just a bit. First, what do we mean by stress, what does it do in the body, and how could it be related to ADHD?

In this context, we are not talking about "good stress" (like falling in love or starting a new job for adults, or an exciting trip or new school year for children) but about "bad stress" like losses, disappointments, or threats. How do we respond biologically and psychologically to stress? A *healthy* stress response means that, given even a bad stressor, we can manage it psychologically. We experience temporary physiological changes when we encounter the stressor, which helps us cope with it, and then we soon return to our own "normal" (called *baseline* or *homeostasis*). In fact, recent research suggests that routine stress to some degree really does make us stronger and more resilient, and even severe stress can be positive if we manage to master it. But a *toxic* stress response occurs when emotional stress cannot be managed, is psychologically overwhelming, or is ongoing and as a result the body remains in an active physiological stress state; see the box on the next page. That's really the concern of this chapter.

A CLOSER LOOK AT TOXIC STRESS REACTION

A toxic stress reaction doesn't mean the stressor is toxic (even less does it mean the person is "toxic"!), but that the body goes into a perpetual stress-response or "ready" state that is unhealthy for the person experiencing it. This happens, for example, to some people who have had a traumatic experience. As a result, people with a history of trauma can react to minor stressors, challenges, or affronts as if they are major threats—with hyperarousal, intense emotion, and difficulty modulating their reaction. Because they have less resilience to stress than other children, kids with ADHD may feel more traumatized by seemingly moderate setbacks and may also end up at times seeming to overreact to acute stress—a single occurrence of a stressor, such as being criticized by a teacher or having a conflict on the playground—as if it's a much more serious threat. But they can also experience chronic "toxic stress" from the fallout of their symptoms: others becoming aggravated by their impulsivity or inattention, feeling constantly off balance or criticized, or being constantly unable to keep up at school, for example. This may build up into a steady state of being overstressed sufficiently to interfere with their self-regulation. Here's part of what's going on in the body when stress reaction is sustained and thus toxic:

- The body secretes more hormones such as cortisol and adrenaline. These are super helpful in an acute threat situation, but if sustained they cause biological damage, for example cell death, and add to a tendency toward intense emotional reactions to even small threats when they are constantly activated. They were designed to activate only sometimes, not continuously.

- The sympathetic and parasympathetic nervous systems go into overdrive.

- The parasympathetic system handles automatic life-support functions, so heart rate may speed up or breathing become more shallow and fast when chronically stress-activated.

- The sympathetic system also adjusts heart rate, breathing, and other responses to help support self-directed efforts at rallying to meet a challenge. It may fail to respond as effectively if constantly challenged by a chronic toxic stress response. This can contribute to failing to modulate one's reaction to an affront that is actually fairly minor.

- The recurrent activation of this system takes a toll on the body and brain that can be measured biologically. This "wear and tear" on the body from chronic emotional stress, called *allostatic load,* is an important concept in today's research.

- Epigenetic changes occur, discussed later in this chapter. Some of these can be in the germ line, that is, can be inherited by offspring and thus cause developmental changes in the next generation.

When a toxic stress response occurs in early life, such as to the mother while pregnant, the fetus detects it through hormonal signals passed though the umbilical cord and placenta. The development of the fetus's brain and other organs changes, leading to changes in future development, temperament, and behavior. When adversity colors the child's development, changes in gene expression and self-regulation also occur. All of this involves epigenetic changes in the developing child's brain, making her more threat-sensitive and thus more reactive to future stress. Scientists have demonstrated this in numerous animal studies, but there is every reason to believe the processes are similar in us. In animals, scientists achieve this knowledge by stressing pregnant rats, for example, by confining them in a tube where they cannot move for a period of time each day or night. This is quite stressful for them, and their bodies react accordingly with hormonal and other physical changes. Offspring are then studied for behavior and growth rate, and their brains are later examined. These studies demonstrate faster physical maturation, bigger behavioral reactions to stress, and stable, epigenetically driven changes in gene expression in the offspring of the stressed animals.

Why does this happen? What is the impact on the child's success in life? One route is actually adaptive—the body, trained by evolution, sets the "thermostat" on self-regulation lower so the child is more reactive. Over the course of evolution, that proved to offer a survival advantage in a very dangerous environment. Very recent research seems to be confirming that when children are in an adverse environment today, they tend to be less regulated, which can still offer an advantage in terms of their chances of surviving or thriving. For example, in a resource-rich environment (like a comfortable suburb), it can really pay off to exert self-control and wait for something good that is promised. But in a resource-poor environment (like a very challenging low-income neighborhood), taking an immediate opportunity instead of something that might pay off later could better promote survival and prosperity, because the future is very uncertain. Thus, if your child is growing up in a very resource-poor or unpredictable environment, her dysregulation or impulsiveness compared to kids from other environments may be nature's way of trying to give her an edge in the environment in which she lives (see the box on the next page).

DOES WEAK SELF-REGULATION ALWAYS WORK AGAINST US?

Evolutionary theory posits that during fetal and early infant develop-ment, our bodies automatically adjust various internal set points to maximize our chances of surviving in the "expected" environment. For example, when a mother is very stressed during pregnancy, the fetus's biology adjusts to an expected adverse world. Scientists have long known that children from lower-income and poor neighbor-hoods seem to be "less regulated" than children from more well-off, middle-class families. A classic way this is tested is by looking at the ability to delay gratification, either on a laboratory test ("If you can resist eating this piece of candy for the next five minutes, you can have two pieces") or in behavior rated by parents and teachers. This may be part of the reason that children from disadvantaged back-grounds are more likely to be identified as having behavior prob-lems, including ADHD.

However, for them apparent impulsivity and emotionality is not necessarily a disorder but can be an adaptation. In a recent study, researchers looked at heart rate adjustment on a measure called respiratory sinus arrhythmia, an index of a biological func-tion called vagal tone. It is thought that vagal tone rises when a regulated, adaptive response is being made. In this experiment, children were asked to delay gratification on a laboratory test. Chil-dren from middle- and upper-class backgrounds showed the famil-iar pattern: when they were able to delay gratification, vagal tone increased. Positive regulation meant positive adaptation. Children from disadvantaged backgrounds, as expected, were more likely to seize the immediate reward and not to delay gratification. However, their vagal tone increased when they did so—suggesting this was the body's adaptive intention, not a failure of regulation. Other research shows that nonhuman primates are the same as people in that they adjust their preference for immediate or delayed rewards based on assessment of which choice will lead to the best long-term gain. The same finding has been seen in foraging birds by ecologists. Finally, there is anecdotal evidence that Special Forces soldiers who seem dysregulated on return from combat ("reactive," "impulsive") are actually those who had naturally learned the positive adaptation of such reactivity in combat after many tours of duty. The definition of positive/adaptive regulation requires careful thought when chil-dren are faced with adverse environments.

REMEMBERED STRESS: WHEN ADAPTATION GOES AWRY

In the past five years it has become clear that true psychological trauma is an important developmental route for the effects of stress on children's problems with self-regulation. Psychological injury from a chronic or toxic stress response is "remembered" in the form of epigenetic marks in the brain and elsewhere in the body. With psychological trauma, the brain also has attempted to adapt and to prepare for a very difficult environment but has not been able to really put it together. The child just has reduced self-control, but it is not actually helpful to him. The epigenetic thermostat governing the biological basis of self-regulation has been set too low, or at least too low for the child's actual context.

This stress, which is "remembered" in the epigenome, takes the form of developmental changes in brain connectivity and organization. The areas of the brain involved include the same regulatory networks that are altered in ADHD. Thus, the brain findings give us a bridge by which we can see a natural link between the toxic stress response (typically in relation to adversity in early life) and a syndrome that at least resembles ADHD and may in some instances be indistinguishable from other routes to ADHD. Keep in mind that these effects don't occur with all children—we always have to consider the context of susceptibility, itself the product of genotype and other aspects of early developmental environment.

Susceptibility varies among children, so not all children exposed to adversity will develop a toxic stress response or end up with ADHD-like symptoms.

At the level of behavior, then, the "toxic stress response" emerges as a loss of self-regulation. This means that the child is emotionally reactive, irritable, has tantrums, or seems emotionally "explosive"; in short, he has frequent difficulty coping, as his now-sensitized brain misreads each new minor stress as if it were a major one. If the child were still in a traumatic situation facing real danger, this response could be protective, but once the trauma is past, or in everyday life, it quickly leads to problematic behavior and can be interpreted by others as ADHD.

Where does this ineffective form of attempted adaptation leave us? Uncertainty remains about the best way to define the syndrome that emerges in children exposed to adversity and the chronic psychological stress that results, but we know it shares with ADHD the characteristic of poor self-regulation of emotions. In cases of mild adversity or stress, or chronic challenges and deprivation, the treatment and help for the resulting ADHD-like picture may be the same as for other kids with ADHD for all practical purposes, perhaps with the exception of extra emphasis on adding social supports. However, for truly traumatic stress (posttraumatic

> *The toxic stress response can leave some children with almost a hair-trigger response to even the smallest stressor, as if they have to be prepared just in case the situation is serious—even though it isn't.*

stress disorder [PTSD]), the game plan is quite different. More on that later in this chapter and in Chapter 8.

ADHD Leads to More Stress and Adversity

So far we've been talking about how early-life stress can lead to a behavioral syndrome a lot like ADHD. In turn, these self-regulation problems tend to expose children to more stress and adversity than other kids: The reactive, immediate-response, or impulsive actions that, if not too extreme, might have saved them from the jaws of a saber-toothed tiger millennia ago (or from attack if their environment really is a war zone) can now land them in trouble at school, cause problems with family and friends, and make it harder to get ahead in the world as they mature.

Keep in mind, however, that this is only part of ADHD. A common misconception is that ADHD is just a style that was adaptive in hunter-gatherer society but is not adaptive in our relatively sedentary urban/

 WANT TO READ MORE ABOUT THE RESEARCH THAT SHOWS THE STORED DAMAGE OF STRESS ON THE BRAIN AND BODY?

Szyf, M., & Bick, J. (2013). DNA methylation: A mechanism for embedding early life experiences in the genome. *Child Development, 84,* 49–57.

Teicher, M. H., & Samson, J. A. (2016). Annual research review: Enduring neurobiological effects of child abuse and neglect. *Journal of Child Psychology and Psychiatry, 57*(3), 241–266.

agricultural world. A subset of individuals do fit that profile and can be effective in active pursuits like hunting, building, and theater, but struggle in a classroom or office. They may have compensating strengths and supports or a relatively mild version of ADHD. But here I'm talking about a more serious developmental overshoot—there has either been too much subtle neural injury, adversity, or genetic mutation, or a combination of these so that a child's dysregulation is not really adaptive in most contexts. As a result, this child too often does not escape from problems but creates them for himself and others—and would probably fall to the same fate even in a hunter-gatherer world. In that case, if he grows up this way, the child needs to pick the right niche in life but also to develop supplemental skills and supports for coping.

The idea that ADHD seems to incline children to experience more ongoing stress is now being confirmed by research. A national survey study of teenage dating violence published in 2015 identified the most at-risk group as girls with ADHD or substance abuse problems. Additional clarity emerged from a major meta-analysis of nearly thirty studies of ADHD and trauma published in 2016; it revealed striking and previously unappreciated findings. Here the types of adversity studied included abuse, neglect, death of a parent, serious physical injury, and severe poverty. The results showed that a child with ADHD gets into trouble more often; *on average kids with ADHD are 60 percent more likely to have a serious adverse experience as a consequence, not a cause, of ADHD.*

ADHD and Stress Sensitivity

But there's another complication—creating that triple whammy mentioned at the beginning of this chapter: children with ADHD, even if they have not had particular adversity, seem to be extra sensitive to stressful environments and experiences. The same 2016 meta-analysis revealed that, faced with a potentially traumatic experience, an individual with ADHD is almost four times as likely to develop PTSD. Put another way, about 3 percent of the general population gets PTSD, but 10–11 percent of kids with ADHD will get PTSD.

Again we come back to self-regulation abilities. Self-regulation is part of how we cope—that's what it's for. Because they have reduced self-regulation, children with ADHD are less able to cope with challenge, regardless of how they got to ADHD. The effects then can become circular—a child who can't cope displays more behavior problems, adding to family or other stress, which in turn feeds the child's stress level and worsens symptoms.

ADHD and stress can interact in a vicious circle, the self-regulation difficulties causing the child to react badly to stress and the child's reactions causing family stress, which in turn increases the child's stress and behavior problems.

Anna, who asked me to evaluate her seven-year-old son, demonstrates why it makes sense to evaluate the role of stress in ADHD and how complicated the issue of cause can be. Anna's son seemed to have ADHD, and her relationship with him was deteriorating. Meanwhile, she was struggling with guilt because she had smoked while pregnant. Her smoking was her way to cope with the severe emotional strain of living with a boyfriend who constantly threatened to beat her. Living in fear for her safety and the safety of the baby, out of work and dependent on her boyfriend for housing, Anna felt trapped. Shortly after the baby was born, she was able to escape the situation, but she still thought her smoking might have caused her child's ADHD.

With a bit of digging, I learned that Anna and her brother both had ADHD, and that her four-year-old, whom she gave birth to her with her very supportive new husband, was showing no signs of ADHD—even though Anna never did quit smoking. I was able to let her know that even though smoking in pregnancy poses many health risks for offspring, its causal effects on ADHD are slight. We know this from recent, clever studies of surrogate pregnancies with and without smoking: women with ADHD tend to smoke more, and that genetic transmission creates an apparent link between smoking and ADHD (although smoking apparently can contribute causally to irritability in a child).

However, severe stress in pregnancy is a different matter, and Anna and I discussed how fortunate it was that she had the courage, resourcefulness, and luck to free herself from her agonizing situation with her partner while pregnant with her first child to find a more stable life with her second.

Stress studies with causal designs in humans are lacking, but as we reviewed in the last section, the data are pointing to where the puck is probably going: it's likely that severe maternal stress while pregnant can contribute to ADHD or ADHD-like symptoms in offspring. In addition, Anna, who has ADHD, may herself be more stress sensitive and experience a greater physiological response to stress than other women. Based on average effects in the population, we might guess that her genetic history of ADHD and her stress during pregnancy could have affected her first child.

But what about after her child was born? Just as the fetus in the womb is influenced by maternal stress, a child exposed to adversity in everyday life can suffer biological changes. This might have been the case with Anna's child before she extricated herself from her relationship with her abusive boyfriend. Discovering which portions of the stress–adversity story seem to fit her situation can lead her to specific steps she can take to minimize stress and resist or overcome adversity to help her child with ADHD. It may even be possible to "erase" some of the biological "memory" stored in the epigenetic signals by whatever adversity occurred during pregnancy or after Anna's child was born, along with the resulting physical and psychological reactions. I have specific practical suggestions that Anna can use, and you can too, in the second half of this chapter. But first, let's explore the role of adversity.

> *Can you erase some of the biological memory of earlier stress to help your child? It's worth a try.*

The Role of Adversity in ADHD

Adversity refers to a mix of moderate and severe experiences that, on a one-time or chronic basis, wear down or injure our coping capacity. The importance of adversity to health has been a major focus of research in recent years, and its frequent absence is now a glaring oversight in our general accounts of ADHD in books and articles. The question for scientists to answer more fully is whether the adversity route to ADHD, and the biological and temperamental development changes associated with adversity, also occur to a notable extent with less severe stressors. A lot

THE ACE STUDY

The Centers for Disease Control and Prevention oversaw one of the largest studies ever conducted of the effect of adverse early experiences on health outcomes. From 1995 to 1997 over 17,000 health maintenance organization (HMO) members from Southern California who were receiving physical exams at the San Diego Kaiser Permanente assessment centers completed confidential surveys regarding their childhood experiences and current health status and behaviors (about 70 percent of those asked agreed to participate). They were then followed up regularly to look at health outcomes. The adverse experience categories looked at were:

- Psychological abuse (often being insulted, put down, sworn at, or being made to feel physically threatened)

- Physical abuse (often pushed, grabbed, shoved, or hit)

- Sexual abuse (unwanted sexual touching, attempted or actual sexual intercourse)

- Substance abuse in the household (such as living with an alcoholic)

- Mental illness in the household (such as a parent or sibling with severe depression)

- Violence between the parents (such as the mother being often slapped or hit)

- Criminal behavior in the household (such as a family member going to prison)

Half the population surveyed endorsed at least one category, most commonly living with a problem drinker; 25 percent endorsed at least two categories. The study has now yielded dozens of findings linking early childhood adverse experiences to elevated rates of practically all noncommunicable health outcomes from high blood pressure to suicide to unintended pregnancy to alcoholism, depression, and mental illness. The pattern is a dose–response relationship. To quote from one of the main publications, "Persons who had experienced four or more categories of childhood exposure, compared to those who had experienced none, had 4- to 12-fold increased health risks for alcoholism, drug abuse, depression, and suicide attempt; a 2- to 4-fold increase in smoking, poor self-rated health, sexually transmitted disease; and a 1.4- to 1.6-fold increase in physical inactivity and severe obesity. The number of categories of adverse childhood exposures showed a graded relationship to the presence of adult diseases including ischemic heart disease, cancer, chronic lung disease, skeletal fractures, and liver disease. The seven categories of adverse childhood experiences were strongly interrelated and persons with multiple categories of childhood exposure were likely to have multiple health risk factors later in life" (the ACE Study, *American Journal of Preventive Medicine*, 1998). The study's weakness is the older age of participants doing the recall (in their fifties on average, recalling their childhood), the reliance on hindsight, which could be colored by current problems, and lack of nationally representative sample. However, its strength is the large population-based sample. Prior to that study little was known about the cumulative health effects of multiple adverse experiences (as opposed to one event such as abuse). The study dramatically changed health care and prevention perspectives. The participants continue to be followed to look at long-term life and health outcomes, and the study spurred better follow-up studies that yielded similar results, as noted in the text.

of light has been shed on this question by some major studies of adversity and its impact on health and development in recent years.

THE ACE STUDY AND FOLLOW-UP STUDIES

The enduring effects of early-life adversity hit the scientific and medical literature in a big, new way with the major ACE (Adverse Childhood Experiences) Study, conducted on a population in California. (See the box on page 172 for a description of the classic study and main findings.)

The first major findings were published in 1998, showing that the more kinds of adverse childhood experiences one recalled, the worse one's health was in adulthood and the greater the chance of mental illness, such as addiction, depression, anxiety disorder, or PTSD. While over half the respondensts had at least one adverse experience, only 6 percent of the population suffered four or more of them. (If you or your child are in that group, you and she have obviously faced extraordinary challenges.) As the number of these experiences rose in childhood, adult health outcomes worsened.

Since then a raft of studies has pursued the power of early adversity

**WANT TO READ MORE ABOUT THE RESEARCH
ON ADVERSITY AND MENTAL HEALTH OUTCOMES?**

The ACE study: Felitti, V. J., Anda, R. F., Nordenberg, D., Williamson, D. F., Spitz, A. M., Edwards, V., et al. (1998). Relationship of childhood abuse and household dysfunction to many of the leading causes of death in adults: The Adverse Childhood Experiences (ACE) Study. *American Journal of Preventive Medicine, 14*(4), 245–258.

The CDC National Survey of Children's Mental Health: Bethell, C. D., Newacheck, P., Hawes, E., & Halfon, N. (2014). *Health Affairs, 33*(12), 2106–2115.

The Boston study adding children's reports: Finkelhor, D., Shattuck, A., Turner, H., & Hamby, S. (2013). Improving the adverse childhood experiences study scale. *Archives of Pediatric and Adolescent Medicine, 167*(1), 70–75.

The Romanian study: Kennedy, M., Kreppner, J., Knights, N., Kumsta, R., Maughan, B., Golm, D., et al. (2016). Early severe institutional deprivation is associated with a persistent variant of adult attention-deficit/hyperactivity disorder. *Journal of Child Psychology and Psychiatry, 57*(10), 1113–1125.

The ADHD and trauma meta-analysis: Spencer, A. E., Faraone, S. V., Bogucki, O. E., Pope, A. L., Uchida, M., Milad, M. R., et al. (2016). Examining the association between posttraumatic stress disorder and attention-deficit/hyperactivity disorder: A systematic review and meta-analysis. *Journal of Clinical Psychiatry, 77*, 72–83.

Likelihood that kids with ADHD experience more stressful events and more PTSD: Biederman, J., et al. (2013). Examining the nature of the comorbidity between pediatric attention deficit/hyperactivity disorder and post-traumatic stress disorder. *Acta Psychiatrica Scandinavica, 128*, 8.

Frequency of overlap of ADHD and PTSD: Kessler, R., et al. (2006). The prevalence and correlates of adult ADHD in the United States: Results from the National Comorbidity Survey Replication. *American Journal of Psychiatry, 163*, 716.

The dating violence study: McCauley, H. L., Breslau, J. A., Saito, N., & Miller, E. (2015). Psychiatric disorders prior to dating initiation and physical dating violence before age 21: Findings from the National Comorbidity Survey Replication (NCS-R). *Social Psychiatry and Psychiatric Epidemiology, 50*(9), 1357–1365.

to influence children's development and in particular the effects on psychological adjustment and psychiatric problems over time via epigenetic change. The list of relevant adverse experiences was recently modified and improved for children by the Centers for Disease Control National Survey of Children's Health, a random, nationally representative telephone sampling of over 90,000 households conducted every five to seven years, most recently in 2011–2012. Here's the list of relevant child adverse experiences in the CDC study.

- Serious economic hardship
- Witnessing or experiencing violence in the neighborhood
- Alcoholism in the home
- Substance abuse in the home
- Domestic violence
- Mental health problems in the home
- Parental divorce
- Loss of parents to death or incarceration
- Social rejection through racial and ethnic discrimination

In that survey, 43 percent of parents reported that the child had at least one adversity, 19 percent reported at least two adversities, and 10 percent reported at least three. As an example, two studies, one published in 2014 and another in 2016, highlight a similar story. Having even one adverse event increased the odds of a physical or emotional condition, and the more events a child experienced, the more likely he was to have had problems with self-regulation of emotion and behavior. If children were subjected to two or more of these adverse experiences, chances of a serious emotional or behavioral problem (including depression, anxiety, anger problems, and behavior problems) doubled (100 percent increased risk); at three or more, chances were quadrupled. While the study design does not rule out genetic effects (parents with mental health problems may be less able to protect their children from adverse experiences), the researchers highlighted the importance of a safe and stable environment for healthy child development.

The frequency of these adverse events in the lives of children with

ADHD in particular was striking. The national survey study found that 7.9 percent of all children have ADHD as identified by a health professional, with parental agreement. Of those, fully 70 percent had at least one of these nine adverse events in the family or life situation.

The more adverse events experienced by a child, the greater the risk of ADHD and other emotional and behavioral problems.

The 2016 meta-analysis of thirty studies mentioned earlier also showed that extreme early adversity is a risk factor for ADHD, tripling the chances of developing the disorder.

There seems to be little doubt that negative life experiences can change the body's stress system and create a toxic or chronic stress response pattern—leading to a negative cycle in which a child who is least able to cope faces ever more adversity. As a result, self-regulation cannot consolidate during development as it normally would. This type of adversity is likely one route to an ADHD syndrome, with potentially different implications for what a child needs compared to other routes to ADHD.

ADDING CHILDREN'S OWN REPORTS OF ADVERSITY: THE BOSTON STUDY

In 2013 researchers in Boston took another look at the ACE list of adverse experiences with an eye to broadening them and also exploring the link between adversity and mental health problems when children's own reports were added (the ACE study was a retrospective study, meaning it asked adults to look back and report on their childhood experiences in hindsight). The Boston team found that predictions of child mental health outcomes almost doubled when the children's reports of the following items were added:

- Peer victimization (assault, physical intimidation, or emotional victimization)
- Parents always arguing (according to child perception)
- Property victimization (experience of a robbery, theft, or vandalism)

- Someone close to the child having a bad accident or illness
- Exposure to community violence (witnessing crime, murder, assault)
- No good friends (child had no "really good friends at school" at the time of the interview)
- Below-average grades (parent reported that the child had "below-average" grades in school)
- Someone close to the child died because of an accident or illness
- Parent lost job (as reported by the child)
- Parent deployed to war zone (for several months or more)
- Natural disaster (child experienced a "very bad fire, flood, tornado, hurricane, earthquake")
- Removed from family (child was "sent or taken away from his or her family for any reason")
- Very overweight (parent reported that the child was "quite a bit overweight")
- Physical disability (parent reported)
- Ever involved in a bad accident
- Neighborhood violence is a "big problem" (asked in the parent interview)
- Homelessness (a period of time when the child's family "had to live on a street or shelter")
- Repeated a grade

The lists of perceived adverse events were getting longer and longer, and many items won't pertain to most parents and their children. But looking at these lists can give you a way to think about your own "stress/ adversity inventory" as you examine just what different contexts may be influencing your child's behavioral, attention, and emotional problems. In Chapter 9, we talk about integrating awareness of key stressors and adversities in your child's life (and your life) into a plan to help your child, along with other tips for building up your child's capacity to overcome ADHD. Depending on her own history and temperament, your child with ADHD may be particularly sensitive to losses, worries, threats, or injuries, so you may find that some of the events on the survey lists seem more important than others. Note that when I say "sensitive" this doesn't mean your child will necessarily worry more about these events (though some kids with ADHD will); the child may simply dysregulate, misbehave, or melt down more in response. By noticing this and realizing that your child with ADHD is more sensitive or responsive to events, you may identify new ways to support him.

SEVERE ADVERSITY AND PERSISTENT ADHD:
THE ROMANIAN STUDY AND OTHERS

One further key source of findings specific to ADHD comes from a unique study of nearly 200 children adopted from Romanian orphanages into England. Those children lived for up to 3½ years in severely deprived conditions in the late 1980s; conditions were so bad that many children died, so this was a truly extreme set of conditions. However, results are illuminating. These toddlers were adopted into homes in England after the fall of the Ceaușescu regime in Romania 1989. They are now young adults.

A series of papers on these Romanian children, the most recent in 2016, have documented that severe emotional and social deprivation in early life can lead to a variant of ADHD. It was striking that compared to children with low levels of deprivation (whose ADHD rates were typical of the general population), the teens in these Romanian orphanage studies were four times more likely to have ADHD, and their ADHD was nine times more likely to persist into adulthood—because these kids who experienced extreme adversity rarely "grew out" of ADHD. Their form of ADHD was not typical; it was complicated by significant social and emotional problems and features similar to autism spectrum disorder. While the severity of that early environment and the particular variation of ADHD they had are unusual, this set of findings does confirm the principle that ADHD can apparently emerge from severe early adversity. We don't know how well this finding extends to less severe kinds of adversity, but everything we know about the biology of stress and adversity points to the probability that milder adversity can be associated with more common forms of ADHD in some instances.

A final acknowledgment: real cultural differences exist between and within ethnic, cultural, and racial groups in most countries; they are certainly complex and multifaceted in the United States. While a full consideration of race and culture is beyond the scope of this discussion, we have to acknowledge that being part of a racial or ethnic minority can complicate the picture related to stress and adversity. See the box below for a partial list of the issues that come into play.

FAQ: HOW DO CULTURE AND RACE AFFECT ADVERSITY AND ADHD?

The studies described earlier in this chapter show that there is little doubt of a connection between ADHD and adversity. Unfortunately, the question of whether (and how) race and culture affect the experience of adversity is very complex. The interplay of race, racism, stereotypes, social disadvantage, adversity, stress, and trauma is poorly understood, and it is critical that we learn more. For parents of children in racial or cultural minorities, the challenges are real. The specific context of race varies from country to country, so it is difficult to generalize, but a few general principles still seem to hold in many settings.

- ADHD occurs at roughly similar rates across cultures, nations, and races, although more data on variation across community, region, and group is sorely needed.
- Minority children and teens, like other disadvantaged kids, have less access to appropriate services.
- A history of racism in some communities can form an obstacle to successful access to services due either to family mistrust or provider lack of understanding.
- Disadvantaged minority communities are exposed to additional risk factors in addition to the measurable effects of prejudice in many settings, creating a vicious cycle in which minority children are seen as underperforming.
- Perceptions of the behavior associated with ADHD vary across race and culture, affecting assessments of children's behavior and the meaning of the behavior.
- Recent research has documented that the existence of stereotypes directly affects stress and performance in children and adults when they face a challenge.

TAKE-HOME POINTS

Adversity and ADHD

Early trauma or adversity, either to the mother while pregnant or to the young child, can alter the development of self-regulation in the child and, if sufficiently severe, contribute to a type of ADHD that may be different in features and severity than other types of ADHD. This proof of principle is consistent with what we know about the biology of stress in early life and increases the likelihood that less extreme adversity can also lead to more common forms of ADHD in some instances. When there is frank trauma, it has to be recognized if you are going to get the right help for your child. Kids with ADHD need special thought on this front for a few reasons.

First, because of their impulsivity and sometimes poor social judgment, kids with ADHD can get themselves into traumatic situations more easily, although it is reassuring that most still avoid this.

Second, because kids with ADHD have weaker emotional regulation and coping strategies, they are more likely to have a worse reaction—even to the level of PTSD.

If you live in circumstances where your child has more risk of encountering something traumatic, or is facing frequent extreme challenges or frequent danger, it might be important for you to try taking some of the action steps suggested in this chapter.

As you can see from the adverse experience lists used by researchers, some of these events are beyond your control (for example, natural disaster). Others are things you can address (like your own depression or conflict and arguing with your child's other parent). Still others may fall in between (like living in a violent or dangerous neighborhood; you may or may not have the resources to move somewhere safer). These effects are not universal—some children are more susceptible or sensitive, partly due to their genetic makeup. Even in the Romanian study, where 20 percent of these children had serious ADHD and others developed autism or other neurodevelopmental problems, some children were basically healthy—they were very resilient.

Part of this susceptibility is in the biology of the body's stress system. This varies based both on genetics and on very early experiences in the womb and after birth. This is why it can be important to protect your child on the other end: boost the factors that can help your child cope better with whatever adversity seems unavoidable. These factors can be the targets of some general action steps:

✓   **AT A GLANCE**

General Action Steps to Help Your Child Deal with Adversity and Stress

Boost coping skills: These include self-talk, planning, strategies, redirecting her attention, taking a break, seeking help, and relaxation strategies.

Reframe the stress as a challenge:* Some research suggests that the body goes into a different, more healthful physical process if we mentally think we are facing a challenge we can handle versus a stressor that might hurt us. This is especially valuable if the stressor really is a challenge and not a threat to the child (like a big test or a new experience).

Reframe stress as beneficial: Some recent work, while preliminary, suggests that our belief about what stress does can affect what it actually does physiologically. If we believe it makes us stronger or that we learn something valuable, it may be to some extent self-fulfilling.

Develop your child's resilience: When your child is healthy and rested, her body naturally maintains its balance against minor stressors because we are designed to absorb a fair amount of stress as part of the daily "cost" of living on this earth and to bounce back from setbacks.

Provide social support: When your child has parents, other family, friends, and possibly professional help who are "in it" with him, he can draw encouragement and solace from them.

Build your child's reserve strength: A healthy self-identity, self-esteem, memory of past successes, knowledge of future relief from present prob-

---

*For more on this interesting idea, see Kelly McGonigal's *The Upside of Stress* (Avery Publishers, 2015). While these ideas are still controversial and in need of more validation, there is initial evidence that they can be helpful.

lems, and mental and physical capacity all help gird your child against daily adversity.

Manage your own stress, using some of the same coping skills: This both models coping for your child and enables you to be available and responsive to your child's need for support.

ADHD: Difficulty Bouncing Back to Baseline after a Setback

Unfortunately, by its nature ADHD makes the return to their own "normal" (baseline, or homeostasis) harder for children to achieve after a challenge or setback. This might be in part due to accumulated wear and tear from stress. A body of work on a concept called *allostatic load* seeks to measure the physical markers of accumulated, chronic stress. Each time the body has to work to return to its preferred baseline state, it is thought to incur a certain cost. While some stress can build up strength, too much chronic stress is thought to create wear and tear on the body's capacity to return to optimal functioning. Whether the difficulty children with ADHD exhibit in recovering from setbacks is related to this idea of allostatic load is not yet settled.

In addition to their weaker self-regulation, each of the supports listed above is often reduced for children with ADHD. This, however, we might be able to do something about.

Coping skills are reduced because children with ADHD lack the same capacity to engage in positive self-talk ("I can handle this; it's no big deal"), to reframe the situation ("In the big picture, nobody will lose a limb here"; "Maybe that other person didn't mean what he said"), or to call up useful strategies ("I better rest up today because tomorrow is a big day"). Their thinking process is less organized due to weak executive functioning, so inner planning and strategies are likewise less organized and effective. Resilience is reduced because the individual with ADHD overreacts mentally, may be less healthy due to impulsive eating or poor sleeping, or may have more frequent stressful conflict with others. Social support is reduced because children with ADHD tend to have fewer friends and to alienate friends and family members. Reserve strength is therefore reduced because self-esteem is lower, self-identity is less well developed, and there are fewer memories of past successes and less confidence in future relief. Overall the individual with ADHD has less capacity to absorb and bounce back from routine stressors. Yet as noted on page 186, you can counteract many of these.

While the literature is small, we see this physiologically when kids with ADHD have an altered physiological response to minor stress challenges (seen in the laboratory by measuring physiological response while a child is watching a cartoon in which characters are sad or worried, or doing mental math while someone watches). Scientists can also formalize this by measuring subjective feelings of stress (self-report) as well as the body's response to stress (for example, changes in secretion of the hormone cortisol into blood or saliva during a stress challenge). We can also test response of the sympathetic nervous system via measures of heart rate. Heart rate is governed by the combined input of sympathetic and parasympathetic signals, but with today's technology we can separate them pretty well.

Our own study found that there were two kinds of physiological response in ADHD. The main group was overaroused in the presence of the emotional cartoon and had an inadequate physiological "balance," or ability to maintain physical homeostasis. A smaller group actually seemed relatively insensitive to emotional challenge—they were physiologically underaroused. (I noted underarousal versus overarousal variations in ADHD in Chapter 1.) The underaroused kids may be a group that parents complain seem not to care about the feelings of others. They likely need extra help learning empathy. But I'm going to focus on the main group, who seem to have difficulty handling even minor challenges. We'll look at adversity and resilience and from there get to a further set of possible action steps.

Resilience to Adversity

We've known for half a century that some children seem "immune" to adversity and others really are hit hard by it. If we could find out what these ingredients of resilience are, maybe we can apply them to protect more kids. Not surprisingly, some of these elements are inborn characteristics that you can't readily alter, such as physical attractiveness, energy level, and the part of intelligence we are born with. The genetic part of the story obviously is beyond our control. But once again, epigenetic effects matter. So a new insight from studies of gene × environment interaction (which we talked about in Chapter 2) as it pertains to genetic × stress effects is helpful. These newer studies look at particular genotypes in the child. For example, one powerful gene is the serotonin receptor gene. It influences the activity of serotonin, a neurotransmitter in the brain that is central to the brain's self-regulation system. These studies find that, depending on genotype, a child is either *sensitive* or *insensitive* to his early environment.

Researchers have chosen a particularly odd metaphor for this: orchids and dandelions. The implication is that an orchid is a "better outcome" than a dandelion. However, an orchid achieves its "better outcome" only under the right conditions. Otherwise it survives less well than a dandelion. A dandelion can't be an orchid, but it does survive better under a wider range of conditions, including harsher conditions.

The significance in children is that in a nurturing environment the child with gene type A will have perhaps better self-regulation, higher IQ, or more success in life than a child with gene type B. But under conditions of adversity, the child with gene type A will have worse self-regulation, lower IQ, or less success in life than the child with gene type B. We aren't ready to do gene testing for clinical purposes. But we can use the principle to recognize that your child's extra sensitivity to adversity may be genetic and that your sensitive child who struggles with challenges may have extra potential given the right niche and the right kind of support.

The literature on resilience is worth noting, even though some of these findings are long-standing. Recent reviews in 2013, 2014, and 2016 highlight that resilience in children is associated with positive bonds with one or more adult caregivers, consistent parenting, positive friendships, and the ability to put a meaning frame on experience, as well as better self-regulation and executive functioning—something we are obviously focused on here. For you as an adult, resilience is enhanced by positive emotions and optimism, active coping (taking action to try to solve problems), getting social support, finding meaning or purpose, altruism (helping others), reappraisal or reframing of events, and facing fears head on.

Basic physical resilience helps too. Eating well, getting sleep, and positive self-talk—some of the factors noted under the general action steps listed earlier—all help. The literature on resilience in children leads me to suggest that even one of the following action steps can add substantially to resilience. (See the box on pages 186–187 for a few additional tips I've found particularly important in my work with families.)

✓   **AT A GLANCE**

Specific Action Steps to Help Build Resilience in Your Child

Give your child the message, in between other moments, or even at moments of doubt, that you have confidence in him, that you trust him, that you believe in him. Even one adult who has complete belief in the child builds resilience. Maintain that positive relationship.

Establish consistency as a parent so your child knows what to expect. If you find this is hard to do, it may be related to your own sense of being overwhelmed and stressed, so attend to your own coping as well.

Protect your child's self-esteem by ensuring positive experiences in one area of her life. This can mean helping your child find a hobby, sport, skill, or activity in which she feels good about herself. All it takes is one activity or area that builds the child's self-esteem. If nothing else, this can come from some one-on-one quality time you spend with her each week doing something you both enjoy—that action, more than any words, gives the self-esteem–boosting message that she is important.

Carry out the sleep, diet, and exercise ideas from other chapters. Physical health provides a big boost to resilience.

Consider religious or spiritual activities. Religious belief and participation has been found to support resilience, in part because it comes with social support, in part because it helps provide meaning and reframing, and for other reasons.

BEYOND THE SCIENCE: A FEW TIPS FOR HELPING YOUR CHILD WITH STRESS

Here are a few extra thoughts beyond what the research indicates, from my own clinical experience with families.

1. **Positive family time with your child can pay huge dividends.** Reserves for handling stress without overreacting can come from building up positive memories, confidence, and hope. Make sure every week to protect some special time where you and your child do something you both enjoy. Give your child plenty of praise. Remember the insight from sports psychology that a criticism or suggestion works best when sandwiched between positive comments.

2. **Provide matter-of-fact *extra* instructions on avoiding traumatic events.** One example is avoiding problems on the Internet, which we touched on in Chapter 5. Others concern playing with guns or knives and meeting unknown adults. Your child's potential for impulsivity, novelty seeking, or emotional misjudgment of a situation exposes her to a lot of risk, but a good deal of it is avoidable.

3. **Supervise your child's social outings from time to time to keep an eye on his social skills and help him improve socially.** It's okay to "coach" your child a bit before the outing, sandwiching suggestions in between praise and encouragement. In particular, if you learn of bullying or other social problems for your child that your child cannot manage even with your coaching, then step in with teachers or other parents to address it.

4. **Very important, and difficult for us all, is to admit you need help, and get it.** If you realize your own history of adverse events is triggering you into frequent putdowns or excessive critical comments to your child, seek professional counseling. In particular, if you find you are overreacting all the time, always angry, or harboring constant negative, resentful thoughts and beliefs about your child, it is a sign that getting your own counseling will be helpful to free you from these preoccupations and make you more mentally and emotionally available to your child.

   Likewise, if you see that a lot of discord is going on between you and a coparent, get counseling. One of the most sobering findings in developmental research is that children very accurately perceive strife between parents—more accurately at times than we adults do ourselves. A striking finding in our own research study is that the child's perception of parental arguing, particularly if it concerns him, is a reliable predictor of the severity of ADHD symptoms observed by the teacher. While we don't know the causal direction here (parents may argue more about a child with more severe problems), part of the link may be the child feeling negatively about himself. So, this is a good one to work with. It takes courage, but the dividends are real. Other family conflicts (such as an overly hostile sibling relationship) may also warrant visiting a pro if it can't be toned down by your own efforts.

Provide motivation—a reason to overcome the challenge, a purpose. Set goals and hopes as reminders.

Cultivate teacher interest in the child. Meet with your child's teacher regularly; help her understand your child; compare notes.

Plan ahead. This is a real weakness for kids with ADHD, so you can help by practicing planning with them, talking to them about plans, and giving them a chance to comment on plans before plans are finalized. If your child is anxious about what is happening, you'll have to frame it accordingly, but here your goal is to reduce the unexpected. You loan the child your executive functions in this sense.

Make sure your child gets the basics of academic skills, especially reading. Invest in that extra reading help to instill the basic ability to read early on.

Make sure your child has at least one good friend—and avoids negative peers. You may have to do some extra coaching or facilitating to assist your child in finding that peer or peer group that she can fit in with. If your child doesn't have a friend, consider a big-brother/sister linkage. See the box on page 188 for more on this important ingredient in resilience.

Teach active coping skills. Help your child learn to reframe the meaning of events, anticipate potentially difficult events, take problem-solving action, and avoid problems. A good counselor will readily be able to work

GETTING SOCIAL SUPPORT

Social support is often the biggest challenge for you and your child if your child has ADHD. When a child has ADHD, entire families can become isolated. Recent studies have documented that stigma is a reality for kids who don't "fit in" or who get labeled as "different" by their social world, including those who have ADHD. For one thing, dealing with your child can be all-consuming so you have less time and less mental space for socializing. For another thing, other families may not want to be around your child because he is so difficult, unpleasant, or annoying to them.

Here, you can attend to your own social support, even if it is only one friend or other couple you can talk to who sympathize, will join you for activities, or share your journey due to their own child's struggles. We list some support groups in the Resources at the back of the book.

For your child, you may have to consider some professional help for social skills training. Many towns have counselors who specialize in social skills groups for children. You may also assist your child by facilitating and supervising play dates.

with your child on coping skills if needed and guide you on tactics for active coping that you can model or encourage for your child.

If you need counseling, consider one of the several new counseling methods focused on building up resilience.

Can the Epigenetic Effects of Stress and Adversity Be Reversed?

Now we come to some good news: new evidence suggests that at least some of the biological and epigenetic effects of stress on development may be reversible with the right environment. The picture is increasingly hopeful, although we have to separate "hype" and "promise" from facts on the ground. First, some of the promise.

A major review of scientific studies in 2014 summarized the animal studies that seek to reverse the neurobiological and epigenetic changes caused by early-life stress in particular (see the box on page 190 if you want to look up the articles that report the research findings). It pointed out three trends:

1. *Scientists have begun to demonstrate in animals that the epigenetic effects of early-life stress can be reversed by injecting certain drugs.* The typical design is to stress the offspring by removing it from its mother (maternal deprivation). When the animal grows up, it is tested for various behaviors such as activity, exploration, and fear reactivity. The animals are randomly assigned to receive an injection of a relevant drug. Their brains are later studied for molecular epigenetic change in key brain regions. An epigenetic signal called histone acetylation is a major focus of these studies because some of the drugs directly target acetylation. These studies show that these drugs can reverse the behavioral effect of early-life stress and do so in part by reversing epigenetic settings in the brain. While we are a long way from human trials that mimic these animal studies, the proof of principle is striking for some of the medications currently in use. Several medications have shown initial promise in animal studies, including anti-inflammatory drugs injected into the brain, drugs that directly affect methylation or acetylation, and some psychiatric drugs such as antidepressants. Their benefits in cases of trauma recovery remain under investigation. Dietary effects via omega-3 supplementation, which has anti-inflammatory properties, may also emerge and need more investigation although benefits are likely to be subtle.

2. *The second conclusion was that high-quality maternal care in early life can reverse the epigenetic effects of prenatal stress on the infant.* One reason seems to be that strong maternal care, touch, and nurturance alter oxytocin production in the infant brain, which in turn changes the epigenetic marks that regulate gene expression in the HPA axis (the body's stress-response system). This provides considerable hope for mothers who had a rough time in pregnancy that their baby can still be protected from adverse effects by a very responsive caregiving approach in early life. In fact, one of the key gaps in studies of ADHD is to what extent extra caregiver changes in the first few months of life can prevent or reduce it. (Most studies of early caregiving in ADHD are with children a bit older, such as preschool.) We and others are undertaking studies now to look at

WANT TO READ MORE ABOUT WHETHER EPIGENETIC CHANGES DUE TO STRESS CAN BE REVERSED?

THE 2014 REVIEW OF ANIMAL STUDIES

Harrison, E. L., & Baune, B. T. (2014). Modulation of early stress-induced neurobiological changes: A review of behavioural and pharmacological interventions in animal models. *Translational Psychiatry, 4*(5), e390.

STUDIES OF DRUGS REVERSING EPIGENETIC EFFECTS

Réus, G. Z., Abelaira, H. M., dos Santos, M. A., Carlessi, A. S., Tomaz, D. B., Neotti, M. V., et al. (2013). Ketamine and imipramine in the nucleus accumbens regulate histone deacetylation induced by maternal deprivation and are critical for associated behaviors. *Behavioural Brain Research, 256,* 451–456.

Moloney, R. D., Stilling, R. M., Dinan, T. G., & Cryan, J. F. (2015). Early-life stress-induced visceral hypersensitivity and anxiety behavior is reversed by histone deacetylase inhibition. *Neurogastroenterogy and Motility, 27*(12), 1831–1836.

EXERCISE REVERSING EPIGENETIC EFFECTS AND PROTECTING AGAINST CURRENT STRESS

Kashimoto, R. K., Toffoli, L. V., Manfredo, M. H., Volpini, V. L., Martins-Pinge, M. C., Pelosi, G. G., et al. (2016). Physical exercise affects the epigenetic programming of rat brain and modulates the adaptive response evoked by repeated restraint stress. *Behavioural Brain Research, 296,* 286–289.

Rodrigues, G. M., Jr., Toffoli, L. V., Manfredo, M. H., Francis-Oliveira, J., Silva, A. S., Raquel, H. A., et al. (2015). Acute stress affects the global DNA methylation profile in rat brain: Modulation by physical exercise. *Behavioural Brain Research, 15*(279), 123–128.

Ieraci A., Mallei, A., Musazzi, L., & Popoli, M. (2015). Physical exercise and acute restraint stress differentially modulate hippocampal brain-derived neurotrophic factor transcripts and epigenetic mechanisms in mice. *Hippocampus, 25*(11), 1380–1392.

whether early-life caregiving is correlated with future ADHD in at-risk babies before attempting intervention studies.

   3. Most hopefully for those already struggling with adversity and ADHD in their child, the benefits of exercise are pretty well established. We touched on this in Chapter 4. However, here I'll add that numerous animal studies have now demonstrated that exercise prior to a stressor specifically protects against the epigenetic effects of stress (by preventing those epigenetic changes) *and* reverses epigenetic changes caused by both early-life stress (modeled by maternal deprivation in rats) and acute stress (modeled by repeatedly restraining the animals).

We can't overstate the positive value of exercise for children who have ADHD or who have suffered adversity or are facing chronic stressors.

Although exercise benefits many systems in the brain, as explained in Chapter 4, the exercise effect is partly understandable because stress and exercise affect expression of a particular gene called BDNF (brain-derived neurotrophic factor) in opposite ways. For example, scientists in Brazil reported in 2015 and 2016 that acute stress (repeated restraint of the animal) triggered multiple molecular epigenetic changes in rats. However, rats that were doing more exercise did not experience the same epigenetic changes. Another report in 2015 from Italy found that the acute effects of stress on the brain's BDNF expression was due to epigenetic changes in the brain. Exercise reversed these effects both in the epigenetic marks and in gene expression. If the effect generalizes to humans, this suggests that exercise can protect against epigenetic changes caused by repeated stress and "heal" stress effects in the brain from both early-life adversity and ongoing childhood adversity including acute extremely stressful events. These benefits may not be total—we don't want to create a false panacea here. But clearly exercise can be one valuable ingredient in helping your child cope better.

Mindfulness: Can It Protect against the Damaging Effects of Stress?

Few solutions to stressful, hyperactive, inattentive modern living are more touted today than the generic domain of "mindfulness." So let's take a look at the theory and the science.

What Is It? Mindfulness means nonjudgmental attention to the present moment. It means being nonjudgmentally aware right now of what is happening around you and what is happening in your own body and mind. A mindful state means I am aware of how I feel, that I am tense or angry or sad, but also that I am aware of what is around me—the other person, the situation. At the same time, I am not judging those observations as good or bad, desirable or undesirable. While I am not "lost in my own head," I also am not reacting to what I notice. Wellness classes typically teach simplified approaches without the religious or philosophical ideas that are related to mindfulness historically. The methods taught in these types of classes include meditation, breath awareness, thought awareness, or movement awareness via exercise like yoga or tai chi.

What Does It Do? Can It Help with ADHD? Can It Help with Managing Stress Reactions? Let me start with the takeaway here: It's becoming clear that mindfulness training doesn't necessarily do much to reduce ADHD symptoms, but it can help you and your child with stress management. I'm going to deemphasize brain effects, for which research is striking but still preliminary, and epigenetic effects because we have no studies for them. Let's move straight to the psychological effects on (1) stress and mood and (2) ADHD itself.

Scientific reviews as recently as 2015 show that acceptance/mindfulness methods, especially if combined with psychotherapy but also in self-help and wellness classes, are somewhat beneficial for difficulties with mood, depression, anxiety, and anger as well as for people who have difficulty coping with stress. One patient summarized the results by saying, "I have the same feelings, but they don't bother me as much." Nearly all of this work was on adults, but some has now been done on children. So this alone may be a reason to consider a wellness class using meditation or some other relaxation and "presence of mind" technique, in view of the minimal risk.

The picture with ADHD symptoms per se, on the other hand, is unconvincing. Since 2008, a handful of studies have looked at whether mindfulness-type practice can help ADHD. Only three studies at this writing have tried to teach children or teens to practice mindfulness. If anything, these findings confirm that these methods do little to help ADHD symptoms but may help associated problems like managing emotions and managing stress in children. One exception may be indirect—

helping with parent stress. A half dozen small studies have tried providing mindfulness training to parent and child together. These showed similar but more encouraging preliminary results in terms of some reduction in ADHD symptoms, probably due to more effective parental presence. On balance, the evidence is too limited to conclude that you should put a huge amount of energy into using this approach to try to make your child's ADHD better directly. Instead, think of it as a tool for stress management that may help your child cope—especially if you as a parent do the same. It may help manage the emotional regulation problems your child is having.

PROFESSIONAL HELP: MINDFULNESS–BASED COGNITIVE THERAPY

The real benefit of mindfulness for mental health and for helping you overcome your own struggle with past trauma or adversity—or trauma's secondary effects on your child's ADHD-related problems with emotional self-regulation—lies with enhanced psychotherapies called "third wave" psychotherapies. These essentially integrate mindfulness practices into a cognitive therapy approach. A particularly interesting example is called, unsurprisingly, mindfulness-based cognitive therapy (MBCT). A 2016 meta-analysis concluded this approach is efficacious for preventing depression relapse. Prior research has suggested it can help alleviate depression as well. A 2016 meta-analysis of ADHD symptoms concluded that MBCT can also help reduce symptoms of inattention, at least in adults, and possibly in adolescents. Overall, this approach enriches the tools available if you or your family are struggling.

Several resources designed for the layperson have been made available by the therapeutic community, tailored in different ways for stress reduction, depression, and other problems. For example, Steven Hayes, an expert therapist, offers a self-help manual that combines cognitive and mindfulness tools for adults, *Get Out of Your Mind and Into Your Life*. Tailored for depression is *The Mindful Way Through Depression*, by John Teasdale, Mark Williams, Zindel Segal, and Jon Kabat-Zinn. It is related to mindfulness-based stress reduction, a method usable via self-help developed by Kabat-Zinn and popularized through his books, such as the book *Wherever You Go, There You Are*. These might be one place to start if you want help in this direction.

WANT TO READ MORE ABOUT MINDFULNESS AND STRESS?

Kallapiran, K., Koo, S., Kirubakaran, R., & Hancock, K. (2015). Effectiveness of mindfulness in improving mental health symptoms of children and adolescents: A meta-analysis. *Child and Adolescent Mental Health, 20,* 182–194.

Kuyken, W., Warren, F. C., Taylor, R. S., Whalley, B., Crane, C., Bondolfi, G., et al. (2016). Efficacy of mindfulness-based cognitive therapy in prevention of depressive relapse: An individual patient data meta-analysis from randomized trials. *JAMA Psychiatry, 73*(6), 565–574.

The takeaway: if you are dealing with your own anger problems including major resentment of your child, finding yourself criticizing your child a lot, or struggling with past trauma or adversity yourself, it's best to see a professional therapist. Tell your therapist why you are there, and the therapist can provide an appropriate psychotherapy that should provide some relief. These updated therapies have good evidence supporting them.

 AT A GLANCE

Action Steps to Get the Help You Need—
Including for Yourself

Pulling apart the ways that stress and adversity might be creating ADHD or ADHD-like symptoms in your child is tricky. Here are some guidelines in summary:

- If your child has experienced adversity or chronic early-life stress, follow the same action plan as you would for ADHD, but don't rely on medication alone. Be sure to consult with a counselor or therapist who can help adjust the action plan if needed and provide help and extra support for coping with stress. Symptoms of PTSD can include being easily startled, having nightmares, and avoiding situations that remind you of the trauma, as well as symptoms of emotional dysregulation that we've talked about.

If you believe it's possible your child has developed PTSD, seek a professional evaluation. PTSD can be mistaken for ADHD, but the professional treatment is quite different. The counselor has to help the child integrate the traumatic experience, and for most children the gold-standard therapy approach is called trauma-focused cognitive-behavioral therapy, or TF-CBT. Very young children may need a variation utilizing parent guidance so you can work with your child. Bottom line: if you suspect a real trauma is involved for your child, get careful diagnosis and appropriately targeted counseling. See the Resources section for where to learn more about different kinds of therapy for trauma recovery for kids and adults.

• Be sure to read Chapter 9, where you'll find a lot more on creating a plan to help your individual child.

• Remember that a child with ADHD really does generate stress in self and others. Parents can become isolated and overwhelmed, generating more stress for the child; and due to impulsivity and poor judgment, children with ADHD are more likely to get into negative experiences. All of this can create a kind of "vicious circle" that you may struggle to identify and try to interrupt. If not addressed, you can end up with something like a traumatizing home environment, where family members are retraumatizing one another. If this is you, know that you are not alone—this kind of dynamic happens to many parents when a child has ADHD, as well as when a family member has been through too much trauma or adversity. It's not your fault, or your child's fault—it's what happens when families are overwhelmed by a special need, event, or circumstance, whether it be a child with ADHD or otherwise. Simply recognize your situation is step 1, and then you can take constructive steps to change it.

1. Recognize that stress and adversity are legitimate targets for you to try to address. Too little emphasis has been placed on the importance of life stressors in terms of both making ADHD worse (or in severe cases, even causing it), and as part of what complicates life for families with ADHD.

2. Know that modern psychotherapies for helping you or your

child cope with stress overload or past trauma are effective and seek them out confidently. If you are overwhelmed by parenting challenges, as many parents of children with ADHD are, parenting counseling can help.

3. You may powerfully protect your child and build her resilience to future adversity just by keeping your home a place of safety and your relationship with your child a sanctuary where your child is safe and supported, in addition to being guided. If you are a new parent, *a hopeful finding is that extra nurturance during infancy can reverse the effects of stress during pregnancy.* The tools from prior chapters, like nutrition, exercise, and sleep, are highly relevant here, with exercise potentially offering particular value. The future may see new medications.

4. The most challenging task is to recognize when you yourself are overwhelmed and need to get professional help for yourself or for your child. If you are carrying your own history of trauma or adversity, be kind to yourself, build up your social supports, and get counseling to strengthen your coping skills.

5. Most of all, be kind to yourself.

8

Getting Professional Help

Traditional and Alternative
Treatments for ADHD

Everything you've read so far in this book should have given you hope that you can help your child by making some adjustments in lifestyle and other factors that are part of the child's ongoing daily experience. I've noted several times, however, that most families who have a child with ADHD will need professional help too. Naturally some of the most frequently asked questions from parents are about what really is the best treatment for ADHD: "How do we know whether our child needs medication, and if we decide to go this route, what are the risks?" "Does behavior management really work?" "How long will it take?" "What kind of support should we expect from the schools?" Unless your child has a very mild case of ADHD, getting the best possible help for your child's symptoms and overall well-being usually involves a combination of measures you can take on your own and treatment and support from professionals. But, of course, it all starts with a proper diagnosis, and there may be more controversy about accurate diagnosis of ADHD than of any other mental health problem. In Chapter 7 I gave one example of the ramifications of an inaccurate diagnosis: a trauma reaction can mimic ADHD at first glance. Yet the proper treatment for a posttraumatic reaction would be very different from the proper treatment for ADHD. Similarly, for a nonspecialist it can be easy to confuse depression, anxiety, or learning disorders with ADHD. Here, too, some of the treatment approaches would be quite different (despite some overlap with the lifestyle suggestions in earlier chapters). So it's important to know what the science tells us belongs in a clinical evaluation for ADHD and related conditions (and what doesn't) and then how to interpret the results.

Standard treatments for ADHD are described in detail in other books (see the Resources). Therefore, I don't delve into them in great depth. Instead, I focus here on briefly consolidating the wealth of studies on ADHD treatment over the past fifteen years and highlighting recent developments. The bottom line is that the workhorses of professional care for ADHD remain parent-based management of child behavior using behavioral strategies, carefully prescribed and monitored medication support with stimulants, and appropriate school planning. However, several controversies in assessment and helpful summations of a decade of complex and nuanced studies can enhance your understanding here. The recent literature enables us to polish our understanding of assessment and treatment, despite no major new developments.

Getting a Professional Evaluation

In Chapter 7 I gave you some red flags that might help you decide whether you need to get professional help for yourself, for the sake of your child. Now we'll come back to getting help directly for your child—although this may also mean beefing up your own skills or supports as a parent.

If your child has enduring problems with some form of self-regulation, and some of the lifestyle and health insights in the prior chapters just aren't cutting it, it's time for a professional evaluation. Here are some signs that it's time.

- My child is falling significantly behind in school because he can't get organized, loses his homework all the time, or just can't stay on task at school.
- My child doesn't seem to have any friends or, worse, is scapegoated or teased because of his behavior.
- My child is demoralized and feels she can't do anything right, and I can't seem to shift this.
- My relationship with my child is in tatters, and I can't get it back on track.

- My child's behavior seems to be dominating our entire family's life, and we cannot get on top of it.

- My child's teachers have expressed ongoing concerns.

At this point it should be clear that children with self-regulation problems vary widely in the expression of those problems, their severity, and the causative factors behind them. There are just too many medical and psychological conditions that can seem like ADHD to try to make your own diagnosis. A trained professional can help you sort out whether your child is dealing with depression, an anxiety disorder, a learning disability, a stress or trauma reaction, a metabolic problem, or a rare or more serious condition such as bipolar disorder, in addition to giving you a clear and detailed picture of your child's self-regulation problems and whether they meet the criteria for ADHD. Armed with the preceding chapters, you'll be able to partner with your child's clinician to look at whether the problems are likely being influenced by your child's sleep, nutrition, or adverse experiences as well.

> *Resist any urge to diagnose your child yourself or to just ask your pediatrician to prescribe medication without a thorough professional evaluation.*

WHAT TO LOOK FOR, WHAT TO EXPECT, AND COMMON MISTAKES DURING ADHD ASSESSMENT

Like most other experts and many parents, I see a typical brief ADHD evaluation in a doctor's office as insufficiently thorough. This is not the doctor's fault—even many pediatricians feel this way. The primary care physician is often obliged by scheduling and contract requirements to fit visits into a structure that isn't suited to a thorough evaluation for ADHD—yet they have no place else to send you. Specialists like me and others are working actively with associations for generalist providers like pediatricians and family practice physicians to try to find more valid, reliable, shorter evaluation and screening tools they can use in that situation. For now, though, the gold standard is still a more detailed evaluation. As a result, often it is necessary to see a child psychiatrist or a child psychologist to get a more detailed evaluation. But in any case, what should you expect? And what are the common mistakes that get people off track?

The scientific literature on ADHD assessment has not changed. It still gives these key messages:

- Essential: standardized, well-normed behavioral ratings instruments.

- Essential: independent information from different observers (such as you and a teacher).

- Essential: clinical judgment. No "pure test" exists. The clinician has to compare what she sees with typical child development, transient problems, and other conditions.

Practice guidelines were promulgated by the American Academy of Child and Adolescent Psychiatry most recently in 2007. I amplify and modify from there based on more recent science and focus most of this section on addressing common questions regarding different elements of professional care.

What a Good Evaluation Should Include—This Has Not Changed

Medical checkup to rule out medical causes of attention problems such as thyroid disease, iron deficiency anemia, infection, sleep disorder (see Chapter 4), or other causes. The skilled physician usually can either rule out these problems or recognize the need for further evaluation once alerted to attention and impulsivity concerns brought up by you, teachers, or others.

Clinical interview to make sure that the problems reported are consistent, have lasted for a long time (rather than having an episodic quality), and that the child is in fact impaired by them (*impaired* means that they are interfering in more than a "typical child" way with important developmental tasks for your child, like school, social development, and family relations). The clinician should make sure a history of adverse experiences or trauma is not being overlooked or misjudged. As I noted, if the real problem is a posttraumatic reaction, the clinical and therapeutic approach is quite different than for ADHD, even though the self-regulation problems might look similar at first glance. The interview process should include observation and interaction with the child. While seasoned clinicians realize that most children don't behave the same in the office as at home, they can notice symptoms and behavior that you may miss—just as you notice things they can't see. Team effort is your watchword.

Standardized behavior rating scales from parent and teacher to see how child behavior fits with national norms and standardized cutoffs and evaluate how much the child's problematic behaviors cross over from situation to situation (such as appearing at home as well as at school). These should be scored and referenced to national norms. Your clinician should be able to tell you what percentile your child scores here, just like for height and weight. Many countries in the world now have at least one nationally normed instrument, although the quality of these varies, and they do not always adequately cover variation based on race or culture.

Child report. Children over the age of eleven should also complete self-ratings of mood and behavior. Younger children have difficulty accurately rating their own experience, although it remains helpful to listen to their concerns and consider their input—doing so gives them a voice, helps us understand specific behaviors, and can also help the child accept the new plans. Self-report of their experience becomes more crucial for older children (after about age eleven). While some children still tend to deny all problems, at this age more children are able to report meaningfully on the degree to which they are troubled or frustrated by not being able to remember, focus, attend, or get motivated—or by worry, depression, peer problems, or other concerns.

In the boxes on the following pages are some questions parents often ask about the diagnostic process.

OUTCOME OF THE EVALUATION

At the end of an evaluation, the clinician should provide you with a summary of the diagnostic picture and a plan for addressing the problem, in language you can understand. Clinical psychologists and neuropsychologists typically provide a written report as well if testing was conducted. You should leave the evaluation knowing clearly what the next step is

FAQ: ARE SPECIAL TESTS WORTH IT?

To assess the usefulness of some of these specific special tests, I'm obliged to refer to my clinical experience due to the absence of research studies on them. But the bottom line is, yes, some additional evaluation is warranted in many cases of possible ADHD. Ancillary evaluations that have been well recognized and for which there is no significant new science to add include:

Neuropsychological Evaluation. While there is no diagnostic test for ADHD, and while consensus guidelines do not recommend neuropsychological testing in all instances, it is helpful in some cases, including when:

- The picture is atypical, unclear, or unusually complex.

- There is a question of unusual or delayed intellectual development, unusual learning style, or learning disability.

- Input is needed on how to design an educational and behavioral program that addresses the child's particular learning profile. (In some instances, an educational psychology evaluation by the school may be sufficient to rule out or identify a learning disability.)

A neuropsychological evaluation can help address some of the individual variations in ADHD, such as whether a child has problems mainly in executive functioning, in focused or divided attention, or in staying alert over time. It can also help determine whether the child learns best through visual or auditory inputs and whether he has difficulty with implicit learning. While not diagnostic, these insights are typically helpful for school planning and sometimes also help you as a parent understand how to get through to your child.

Speech and Language Evaluation. If your child has speech or communication delays, this may be an important evaluation. A receptive language disorder can mimic an attention disorder at first glance. A language delay, while not likely to be confused with ADHD, can occur with ADHD.

Occupational Therapy. An evaluation by an occupational therapist can be valuable if your child has noticeable fine-motor delays (learning to tie shoes or button clothes; struggling with handwriting) or gross-motor delays (clumsy, uncoordinated).

Hearing Evaluation. Hearing is often screened at school or the doctor's office. A routine hearing evaluation should be conducted to ensure that

Carefully consider additional testing for your child based on your child's individual profile that emerges from the evaluation.

listening and hearing are normal. See the information below about central auditory processing.

Ophthalmology. Proper randomized studies to evaluate the overlap of eye problems and ADHD are lacking, and the few careful case control and clinical studies in recent years have yielded mixed results—but this mix may be enough to raise concerns. One anecdotal case I saw underscores the issue. Nine-year-old Cecil was referred for psychological testing to address inattention, lack of focus, and learning problems in school. The school had tested his reading and found he had a grade-level reading score. The test results were unusual: Cecil had normal verbal intelligence, but the nonverbal tests showed an unusual pattern. His reading scores were at grade level, but qualitatively, reading was effortful and taxing. Cecil avoided reading and could not remember what he read. He was referred for a detailed eye exam, which yielded several abnormal findings related to poor eye muscle control and coordination (poor near-point convergence and tracking and weak binocularity—the ability to use the two eyes together). His learning problems were "cured" after treatment for the vision problems.

While it's not part of the psychiatry guidelines, one very recent analysis in the medical ophthalmology literature suggests that it is prudent to have a complete eye exam if ADHD or learning problems are not responding well to treatment and particularly if there is difficulty focusing when reading or writing. Although rare, ocular issues such as accommodation, ocular motility, and binocular function (especially near-point convergence) and high refractive errors could mimic a reading or attention problem.

Other High-Tech Evaluation and Treatment Tools. Several new tech-based evaluation options have come on the market. The bottom line is that all of these can be safely skipped. Each remains expensive and either lacks adequate validation data to justify the expense or is unproven. Because you will run into strong claims for the value of these options, I include the latest updates in the box on pages 204–206, along with information on further reading if you're interested. I touched on high-tech treatments in Chapter 5 as well.

At the time of this writing, we don't have the data to suggest that the new, often high-tech assessment options are worth the expense.

**UPDATE ON THE LATEST TESTS:
NOT WORTH THE EXPENSE**

EEG Brain Wave Testing. Recently the FDA approved an EEG evaluation that uses slow-wave brain signals as an aid to ADHD diagnosis. The specific claim is that although the device cannot diagnose ADHD, it can help a clinician identify cases in which the ADHD symptoms may be due to another condition (such as an emotional issue). A study partially funded by the company (NEBA Health) concluded that it could do so. An editorial exchange in the literature in 2016 highlighted the concerns that remain. A team of EEG neuroscientists pointed out methodological weaknesses in the FDA's approval data, including the fact that it did not use the formal diagnostic criteria or replicate the claim of improved rule-out of false-positive cases. Overall, while the direction of this development is promising, use of the EEG test in clinical evaluation is premature. I do not recommend investing in it at this time. This may change as better validation tests are conducted.

Brain Imaging. Some books and publicity have suggested that different kinds of brain imaging can diagnose ADHD. These lack scientific validation. There is no brain imaging test for ADHD that is recognized or supported by published scientific literature. I do not recommend spending your money on these evaluations without a medical justification.

Central Auditory Processing. Some people are interested in a particular condition called a central auditory processing disorder (CAPD). Given the frequency of questions about it and its relative neglect in many ADHD primers, I include a bit more overview here. Some research does show that children with ADHD have particular problems with the brain's electrical response to auditory information, perhaps as a function of the cortex or even at the lower brainstem or sensory levels. A small but fascinating set of studies claim that white noise may improve attentional focus in some children with ADHD. Further, many children with ADHD have a history of ear infections, which if they persist early in development conceivably could interfere with the brain's experience-dependent development of auditory processing. Finally, there is a body of research looking at brain electrical recordings called cortical evoked potentials and brain-stem evoked potentials in relation to problems with hearing. Findings related to autism and auditory processing are also intriguing. At least six sets of clinical guidelines for evaluating central auditory processing using brain electrical recordings now exist (three in the United States, two in Britain, and one in Canada); a recent review praised the guidelines in Britain but noted that even these are not recommended for use without modification. Australia has national evaluation centers that evaluate hearing coordination across the two ears in relation to listening problems with some promise for identifying children who can benefit from specific hearing-listening-related intervention.

However, despite these intriguing leads and reasonable logic, the scientific and clinical literature provides very little validation for a central auditory processing disorder approach to ADHD and insufficient confirmation that an evoked potential measure can be used reliably to diagnose a treatable condition. The main problem, as outlined in a comprehensive review of this area published in 2015 in the *American Journal of Audiology* is that common clinical evaluation tests for CAPD are largely invalid (heavily influenced by attention and executive function rather than hearing tests), so that children with ADHD often test positive for CAPD simply due to having poor executive function. Further, while the ideal would therefore be to rely on brain recordings (ERP measures of auditory evoked responses), here consensus diagnostic standards are lacking and there is no agreed-on clinical protocol for using ERP measures to assess CAPD in ADHD. The expert review did not recommend use of CAPD protocols. Overall, special CAPD testing is generally unjustified if your child has had a competent speech and language evaluation and audiology exam.

Laboratory Tests of Attention and Activity. Numerous measures have been proposed that measure attention in the clinic, such as the Conners Continuous Performance Test, the Test of Variables of Attention (TOVA), and the Integrated Visual and Auditory Continuous Performance Test (IVA CPT), some of which have national norms that can be helpful. Other tools combine such attention tests with motion sensors using infrared sensors or pressure plates, such as the Quotient ADHD System and the Swedish Quantified Behavior Test (QbTest) Plus. These types of tests have a long history, and some of them have obtained FDA approval (which only means they are safe, not that they effective), although currently there are no national norms that would make them truly useful in clinics. While some clinicians find them helpful, and insurance companies will sometimes pay for the test, none of these tests are diagnostic in themselves and their added cost–benefit value is still debated.

Genetic Testing. Several genes have been identified that are related to ADHD, and rare mutations are starting to be discovered that may cause

ADHD. I will not be surprised to see a day arrive in the future when genetic testing is appropriate for children with ADHD. But we aren't there yet. Identification of known genes in your child is unlikely, and even if it happened, it would be insufficient for a diagnosis and would have no effect on treatment recommendations. While this area is rapidly changing, as of 2016 genetic testing is not a useful investment of time or money in the absence of medical indicators for a known genetic or chromosomal condition.

WANT TO READ MORE ABOUT THE DEBATES OVER THE FDA-APPROVED EEG BRAIN WAVE TEST?

Snyder, S. M., Rugino, T. A., Hornig, M., & Stein, M. A. (2015). Integration of an EEG biomarker with a clinician's ADHD evaluation. *Brain and Behavior, 5*(4), e00330.

Arns, M., Loo, S. K., Sterman, M. B., Heinrich, H., Kuntsi, J., Asherson, P., et al. (2016). Editorial perspective: How should child psychologists and psychiatrists interpret FDA device approval? Caveat emptor. *Journal of Child Psychology and Psychiatry, 57*(5), 656–658.

Stein, M. A., Snyder, S. M., Rugino, T. A., & Hornig, M. (2016). Commentary: Objective aids for the assessment of ADHD—further clarification of what FDA approval for marketing means and why NEBA might help clinicians. A response to Arns et al. (2016). *Journal of Child Psychology and Psychiatry, 57*(6), 770–771.

WANT TO READ MORE ABOUT THE POSSIBLE AUDITORY PROCESSING CONNECTION IN ADHD?

Cheng, C. H., Chan, P. Y., Hsieh, Y. W., & Chen, K. F. (2016). A meta-analysis of mismatch negativity in children with attention deficit-hyperactivity disorders. *Neuroscience Letters, 612*, 132–137.

and what to expect. What might be recommended? Let's move on to standard treatments and review the latest.

Treatments

The classic study of treatment for ADHD is called the Multimodal Treatment Study of ADHD, or the MTA study for short. Most of you have probably heard about the initial findings of this study from other books, as the study's initial results were first disseminated in 1999. In subsequent years, follow-up studies of the participating children examined various moderators—characteristics that qualified earlier findings, as well as durability of effects. This major study was conducted at several centers around the United States in the late 1990s, with boys ages seven to nine. After more than a year of treatment, children were followed to early adulthood. Scientific findings on this group have followed as the children are tracked through development. While no new major findings have emerged in the past five years, the dozens of papers from this project have left many parents and clinicians with a somewhat fragmented view of the rich array of nuanced recommendations that emerged. These were helpfully summed up by the MTA team in 2015, and I've listed them in the box on page 208. While not new, these findings may not be widely appreciated.

The crucial point for most of you is that, unless your child has an anxiety condition along with ADHD, combining medication and psychosocial treatment is the best move to maximize chances of positive

---

FAQ: WE HAD AN EVALUATION OF OUR CHILD FOR ADHD AND WERE TOLD THAT DESPITE HAVING SYMPTOMS, HE DOESN'T MEET THE CRITERIA FOR THE DIAGNOSIS. WHAT DO WE DO NOW? WE ARE VERY WORRIED ABOUT HIM. CAN WE STILL GET HELP?

This sometimes happens. In some instances it is an indication that the right course of action is just "wait and see" because your child's problems remain within the variation of typical development or may prove temporary. You may be able to worry less and give it some time. In other cases, this result may mean the child doesn't meet the formal criteria, but the child can still be experiencing interference in life activities and development. This is consistent with the literature that shows even children with "subthreshold" symptoms can be *impaired* (again, that just is a word for real interference in development or everyday activities) by those symptoms. In these cases, the clinician can diagnose *not-otherwise-specified* ADHD, which can justify some professional intervention. In either case, you may still see benefits from the lifestyle changes reviewed in Chapters 3–7. Remember, ADHD may occur on the far end of a trait spectrum from very good self-regulation to very poor self-regulation.

THE MTA STUDY: A COMPREHENSIVE SUMMARY OF FIFTEEN YEARS OF PAPERS

The MTA study sample was all boys ages seven to nine who have now reached early adulthood. Dozens of papers over two decades provide a wealth of fine-grained interpretation for professionals to use. Here are the compilations. These recommendations assume that (1) medication management with stimulants entails frequent (at least monthly) visits to the prescribing clinician to check on symptoms and side effects and carefully adjust dosages, (2) parent counseling uses demonstrated effective methods, and (3) specific stressors such as trauma, a specific learning disability, or medical conditions are appropriately addressed. Here are the take-home points:

- Medication effectiveness requires intensive medical management and dosage adjustment (frequent meetings with the prescriber).

- Highest chances of improvement for ADHD overall: combined treatments, but this depended on parental adjustment of discipline practices with medication effect.

- For ADHD plus anxiety disorder without disruptive behavior: try behavioral counseling alone.

- When parents could reduce negative discipline under professional guidance, children in combined treatment reached normal levels of ADHD symptoms.

- Improving children's social skills helped predict symptom normalization as well.

The one relatively new discovery in the past five years is that treatment gains were not sustained even under routine care in the community. Thus, your child's ultimate benefit from traditional care likely may depend upon ongoing vigilance and periodic return to treatment, even if you obtain a positive initial response.

WANT TO READ MORE?

Hinshaw, S. P., Arnold, L. E., & MTA Cooperative Group. (2015). Attention-deficit hyperactivity disorder, multimodal treatment, and longitudinal outcome: Evidence, paradox, and challenge. *Wiley Interdisciplinary Reviews: Cognitive Science, 6*(1), 39–52.

effects. Also, the child's medication should be managed more intensively than is often the case, through frequent meetings with the doctor and careful adjustment of dosage. It's also important to shift gears in parental discipline to respond to the ways that your child's behavior improves due to the medication. The single most significant parental change in successful outcomes in the MTA study was to reduce negative responses to the child's behavior (a natural response sometimes, but one that is not usually helpful). Overall, it remains most advantageous to combine carefully managed stimulant medication treatment with behavioral methods that you as a parent learn with a counselor and work on at home with your child—along with appropriate school planning.

BEHAVIORAL OR PSYCHOLOGICAL TREATMENTS

Behavioral treatments come in many forms and continue to be refined. While it's tempting to wish for a "major breakthrough" in traditional treatments in light of all that's being learned about ADHD, self-regulation, and epigenetics, much of the mainstream treatment options remain the tried-and-true workhorses. However, a few words on behavioral and psychological treatments are important here because without these, your other efforts are less likely to pay off.

The main news from updated meta-analysis studies in the past couple of years is that behavioral parent guidance or parent counseling is effective for improving your parenting skills and helping with ancillary symptoms like defiance, tantrums, poor social skills, and uncooperative behavior. It can help you teach your child the skills necessary for maturing into sufficient self-regulation. However, it is not clear these psychosocial treatments are very powerful in addressing ADHD symptoms themselves unless combined with medication (although another review disputes this). According to the most recent comprehensive review, parents and teachers do perceive improvement in ADHD symptoms, but this is partly due to expectations; raters who are not aware of the treatment don't reliably see this—but do see the *other* improvements. It may be that because the child's overall attitude and behavior are improved, parents and teachers feel like ADHD symptoms are improved too. Overall, the real focus of these behavioral treatments is on functional improvement (actually doing better in coping with life's problems) rather than symptoms per se. That's pretty important and makes these treatments well worth it.

The most well-established method for behavioral management of children with behavioral and emotional problems involves you, the parent, going to counseling, which is more important for you than for your child. At first this may seem counterintuitive. It's true that many children also need to see a therapist to strengthen their coping and self-management skills, especially if they have mood or anxiety problems. But it makes sense that you have to do the heavy lifting. You are around your child dozens of hours per week. You have thousands of small interactions with your child. A therapist, by contrast, can see your child only for an hour each week in an artificial environment, with only a few interactions. You, the parent, have far greater leverage and influence in helping your child learn to manage his behavior than a therapist ever could. So it actually makes sense that the most effective method is for the therapist to teach you how to work at home with your child. See the box on the facing page for a list of the basic ingredients in parent training.

You and I both know that you know how to be a parent. Many of you are doing just fine with your other children. Our own studies and others showed years ago that most parents of kids with ADHD are normal in their personality, parenting skills, and behaviors (although many get pulled into exchanges with an ADHD child that, if not corrected, can become quite negative, prevent improvement, or even become part of a downward spiral of child problems). But parents of kids with ADHD, like teachers and other caregivers, often don't engage in the most appropriate parenting behavior with them because the child is too provocative and difficult. The adult's skills and capabilities are overloaded and break down. This is another way of recognizing that your child has special needs, and so naturally you need special skills. Now, your child may still benefit from going to counseling too, focused on helping her solve problems, connect actions and results, and interact with caregivers, as well as cope with feeling overwhelmed. If the child

Special needs require special skills.

has an anxiety disorder, she can benefit from individual counseling using a cognitive-behavioral therapy approach. But the main engine of change for kids with ADHD will be your skill building in working with your child as a parent.

BASIC ELEMENTS OF PARENT–BASED TRAINING FOR ADHD

- Ten to twelve sessions of one to two hours (fewer in some group based curricula)

- Education about the nature of ADHD or about family systems, depending on the model

- Identifying the primary problem you want to focus on (start with a specific focus)

- Attending skills (learning to track child's behavior and misbehavior patterns)

- A behavior plan or token economy at home

- Effective use of time-out

- Practicing or teaching relevant skills

- Handling misbehavior in public settings

- Use a daily school report card to track school progress and behavior and coordinate with teacher

- Anticipating and planning for future behavior problems with a planned response (avoiding reactivity)

- Booster sessions

One of the most useful aspects of parent training is learning not to react on autopilot to frustrating behavior.

WANT TO READ MORE ABOUT THE RESEARCH ON PARENT TRAINING PROGRAMS?

Pfiffner, L. J., & Haack, L. M. (2014). Behavior management for school-aged children with ADHD. *Child and Adolescent Psychiatric Clinics of North America, 23*(4), 731–746.

Ollendick, T. H., Greene, R. W., Austin, K. E., Fraire, M. G., Halldorsdottir, T., Allen, K. B., et al. (2016). Parent Management Training and Collaborative & Proactive Solutions: A randomized control trial for oppositional youth. *Journal of Clinical Child and Adolescent Psychology, 45*(5), 591–604.

FAQ: WHAT WILL I LEARN IF I GO TO COUNSELING?

You will learn specific skills to help your interactions with your child get unstuck and move in a positive direction. Which specific skills depends on the approach chosen by your counselor. Based on an expert summary in 2014, two main approaches seem to be about equally effective on average, and the best approach will depend on your existing style and strengths, and the specific profile of your child that you will talk about with your clinician. Each approach can be done either with or without your child present, although progress is sometimes faster with your child present. The text outlines the main approaches. Ask your counselor if he can follow one of these effective approaches with you.

Parent Management Training

The workhorse method is called *parent management training*. This approach is the most established and studied. It derives from behavioral psychology. It was first developed by Connie Hanf at Oregon Health & Science University in the 1960s by consolidating a number of ideas that existed at that time. It has since has been heavily studied, validated, improved on, systematized, and taught in related forms by her former students who are now leaders in the field—Rex Forehand, Russell Barkley, Sheila Eyberg, and others, as well as their students in turn. The assumption here is that the child has learned a negative behavior and needs a motivational structure to help her practice and learn alternative behaviors. This approach focuses on clear expectations, effective communication, and clear, reliable consequences for both positive and negative behavior. Often a point system of some kind is used to help the child see his progress on a frequent basis. These approaches can be very helpful at overcoming a child's noncompliance or being "stuck" in not listening to parent requests. This method is used in Russell Barkley's book for parents, *Taking Charge of ADHD*.

This approach has long been well supported in multiple clinical trials and was the main approach in the MTA study. It is most effective for managing disruptive behaviors and, unless combined with medication treatment, less effective for ADHD symptoms per se. For ADHD symptoms, the little-appreciated but key benefit in the MTA study (shown over a decade ago; see the box on page 208) was that by having a clear strategy, parents were able to reduce negative criticism and arguments with children and become more effective, multiplying the effects of medication.

A related approach, slightly changed to focus almost exclusively on using reward to support the behavior you want, is outlined in an accessible work by parent management training (PMT) expert Alan Kazdin (*The Kazdin Method for Parenting the Defiant Child*). While there aren't specific studies on his method, it uses all the principles of PMT and is well grounded in the literature, including his own studies of PMT. You may use a star chart or point system to "shape" the child's behavior toward the response that you want. A good deal of teaching and practicing is employed. After a response is practiced enough it becomes a habit, and the supportive star chart will no longer be needed.

Collaborative Problem Solving

The second approach is called either collaborative problem solving or collaborative and proactive solutions, depending on whether the particular trainer was from the Harvard/Massachusetts General or the Virginia Tech group. This approach is also called *parent emotion coaching*. It's based on systems principles and skills building. It utilizes dialogue, negotiation, and empowerment in relation to your child. The logic is that a collaborative dialogue can resolve conflict. It was developed by Ross Greene at Virginia Tech University during the 1980s and 1990s, building on earlier work in this vein. This approach assumes that children lack the skills to perform the behavior they need to use. A collaborative approach enables you to teach the child. Despite substantial work disseminated in Dr. Greene's books, until recently it has lacked peer-reviewed studies supporting its effectiveness. However, that is changing with publication in 2015 and 2016 of proper randomized trials. The group has more papers forthcoming. While this literature is therefore still rather thin compared to the literature for PMT, their primary randomized study was well done and showed that PMT and CPS were equivalent, with a 50 percent success rate in normalizing behavior problems. Replication will be needed,

---

FAQ: AM I BRIBING MY CHILD WITH REWARDS?

This is a danger if PMT is not done correctly; in fact there is a literature on how the wrong kind of external reward actually ruins internal motivation. This is actually one of the problems with overly harsh discipline as well—the child complies because of compelling externals, rather than developing internalized control. However, when followed correctly to focus on teaching a particular behavior, a reward system avoids the "reward/bribe" trap. In practical terms in managing children, the main danger comes when a parent starts to "pay" a child with points or rewards for everything ("I'll give you five points to take out the recycling") even when something is not part of the focused plan. Soon the entire relationship becomes transactional. The focus has to remain on helping the child practice a new behavior or skill for a period of time ("Remember, if you can get ready for bed without help again tonight, you get five more points; otherwise we'll try again tomorrow"), not talking him into compliance or into doing the parent a favor at a given moment.

---

but I am hopeful this approach will prove a good alternative for some families. The approach can be looked at on websites at Virginia Tech (*www.livesinthebalance.org*) and Massachusetts General (*www.thinkkids. org*).

FAQ: IF I ENGAGE IN A PROBLEM-SOLVING DISCUSSION WITH MY CHILD, WILL I LOSE MY PARENTING AUTHORITY?

This, too, is a danger that emerges if PMT or collaborative problem solving is not done correctly. The main danger here is that discussions get too involved in a negotiation and trail off into a lost focus, or a request or command is never actually resolved. But this is avoided with the right balance in the approach, with the focus remaining on the problem and on guiding the child toward finding a solution to it. Discuss these worries with your counselor when you start the work; the point of the targeted skills you will learn is to know how to get the results without hitting these traps. Note that it's valuable to explain to the child what you are doing and why. But the explanation should be brief and not turn into a philosophical treatise.

FAQ: WHAT QUALIFICATIONS SHOULD I LOOK FOR IN A COUNSELOR?

Qualifications vary from country to country. In some still-developing countries, the only counselors available have a bachelor's degree. However, in the United States, Canada, Europe, Japan, the United Kingdom, New Zealand, Australia, Ireland, and many other countries, counselors should have an advanced degree (MA, MS, MD, or PhD) and a license. Licenses are granted state by state, so the counselor's office should have displayed in view her state license to practice. Usually, her degree will be displayed as well as other credentials. The degree and license may be any of the following in addition to the licensure/certification:

- Master's in social work (MSW) and license in social work
- Master's in counseling with appropriate counseling license
- Doctorate (PhD) in clinical or counseling psychology
- MD with appropriate background, residency/fellowship, and licensure or certification

If the counselor has the appropriate credentials and experience with your type of situation, is familiar with the various programs for parents of difficult-to-manage children, and is comfortable with the expectations outlined here, you should be on solid ground.

Executive Function Coaching or Organizational Training

This is an area with promising new developments in recent years. The terms *organizational skills training, executive function coaching,* and *ADHD coaching* are somewhat interchangeable. However, they do not always connote a scientifically valid method. Many ADHD coaching systems are "seat of the pants," and not proven programs. It is really only very recently that we have had initial studies that actually demonstrate effective progress for children and teens using a coaching method. So is a good ADHD coach a valid intervention for ADHD? I'd say this intervention falls somewhere in the category of possibly to probably efficacious. We have now seen promising, properly conducted trials that suggest these methods are worth trying—but be aware that the well-done studies have used either professional therapists or school counselors to teach organizational skills. To get to the gold standard, these methods will need additional trials by different independent groups, which have to appear. But the puck seems to be going this way, to recall our hockey metaphor. Critical caveat: Select a properly designed program; there are many untested variations. Note that the focus here is to help with disorganization and time management, not behavioral compliance or hyperactivity. Thus, these approaches are a complement, not a substitute, for other parenting approaches.

Three notable approaches are:

1. *Self-help: Smart but Scattered.* In this program, psychologists Peg Dawson and Richard Guare help parents identify the specific executive functions that are weak and then give them instructions for helping the child acquire new skills and compensate for the weakness by using skills in areas where the child is strong. They also help parents modify the child's environment to reduce dependence on weak skills. While there is no specific clinical trial of this approach, the tools are all sound, low risk, and sensible.

2. *Therapist guided: Organizational Skills Training* (OST). This program was developed by Howard Abikoff, Richard Gallagher, and colleagues in New York. Abikoff is one of the all-time leaders in developing programs for kids with ADHD and evaluating behavioral treatments. A book on OST designed for parents will be available soon after this book is published. OST divides the organizational problems that children with ADHD tend to have into four skill areas and gives them a systematic way to learn, step by step, how to get and stay organized. This is a clinician-administered program, although the therapist builds in meetings with the teacher. The program was developed mainly to help with school success but works for organizational tasks at home as well. One of its keys is that it calls ADHD symptoms "glitches" that interfere with children's potential "mastermind," a feature that apparently helps children depersonalize their symptoms and take on the training without feeling shame or blame for their struggles with ADHD. The authors' first randomized trial, published in 2013, found that just over half the children with ADHD were able to normalize their organizational and time management skills by the end of treatment and one year later retained an improved school attitude and organizational skills at home. A related, school counselor-

based approach for middle school students called HOPS is reviewed in the section below on School-Based Interventions.

3. *Home and school collaborative life skills program.* This program, which emphasizes home–school collaboration, was developed by Linda Pfiffner and colleagues in San Francisco. It combines parent management training (a twelve-week group), school programming, and a child group. Their initial clinical trials published in 2013 showed improvement in both academic functioning and ADHD symptoms as well as organizational skills. A variant of this approach (called child life and attention skills, or CLAS) is less intensive and also showed improvement in ADHD symptoms and organizational skills in a trial published in 2014. School-based mental-health professionals were the primary providers, making this model one that requires school collaboration but that can be set up within schools or school districts, perhaps with a better cost–benefit ratio than other approaches to children with ADHD. It suggests that progress is continuing on effective help for kids with ADHD.

I consider a fourth, school-based approach in the section below on School-Based Interventions. While these programs haven't yet reached the highest level of proof (multiple replicated, double-blind, randomized clinical trials with medium or large effect size), we can see where the puck is going on this one. Many children with ADHD are likely to benefit from organizational skills training or executive function coaching if properly administered, perhaps combined with parent management training and some teacher consultation. The key seems to be the right curriculum and effective engagement and motivation of the child, which these programs try to build in.

The Basic Concept in Organizational Training. The concept here is direct instruction—teaching children and giving them tools to learn how to get organized. In many respects, the tools are the same ones that adults can use to get their own lives organized. It's just that a child who has ADHD needs explicit help staying on track with teaching and focused use of these tools.

The Key Ingredients. The successful programs combined a behavioral program (such as rewards or points for engaging the program) with teaching organizational skills. For some motivated children, the behavioral portion may not be needed, but in general this will greatly increase success. For example, OST (the program from Abikoff and colleagues) proposes twenty sessions on four major topics:

- Tracking assignments (for example, using a daily assignment record)

- Managing materials (school, papers, assignments, backpack checklist)

- Time management (short-term management, long-term planning)

- Task planning (fitting steps, tracking, materials into schedule, long term)

These programs include ample handouts, assignments, and guide materials to help a child develop organizational skills and to help you as a parent guide the child at home and check on progress with the school. Expect quite a bit of structure and quite a bit of activity, but also expect some good results helping your child's problems with being organized and keeping his "stuff" together. The goal here is to build toward independence, so this type of program is often very helpful in middle and high school, when teens struggling with ADHD really need to start getting a handle on these issues as they prepare to grow up and move out into the world.

How to Find a Good Coach. This area is unlicensed and unregulated, although that is rapidly changing. For now, you have to carefully vet your prospective ADHD coach. But good coaches are out there. Look for the following: They should show you their curriculum and materials, point to evidence of success (preferably by pointing to one of the published programs), and have a plan for working with you on child engagement and motivation. Finally, a good coach will know how to coordinate home and school; many coaches I have found doing good work are former special education teachers or otherwise have excellent backgrounds for this type of work. Ask to see the curriculum, ask how progress will be monitored, and ask how the school and you will be involved to support the child's efforts.

Metacognitive Training in School. When the problem relates to executive functioning or organization, special education teachers can often deliver metacognitive skills training. This is related to organizational skills training but is more focused specifically on study habits, study skills, and problem solving. A fundamental question such a teacher might ask a child is "What do you do when you don't know what to do?" From here, the teacher helps the child "think about thinking" and step outside the situation to look at how to create a better situation. Similarly, an older child might be taught how to approach reading assignments with a focus on first identifying "Why am I reading this?" and "What do I want to learn here?" Then strategies for maximizing comprehension are added to the picture. If the child is struggling with concepts, comprehension, organization, or forgetting, then metacognitive training is often a useful part of the educational program and pairs well with an organizational skills coaching treatment.

SCHOOL-BASED INTERVENTIONS

If your child has ADHD, it is advisable to create a collaborative educational program. Under organizational skills I noted one approach that while school based is really focused on the child's skills. Here I discuss more comprehensive programs that school personnel can consider for helping children develop self-regulation, including children with ADHD. A good special education teacher can design a program that can be implemented in the regular classroom once the child's profile is well understood. School-based interventions to assist children with ADHD continue to be refined; in 2014, 2015, and 2016 major syntheses of this literature were offered. Interventions for elementary school children have been studied for quite some time. While recent literature mostly confirms prior findings, a new development in the past five to

 WANT TO READ MORE ABOUT BEHAVIORAL PROGRAMS AND EXECUTIVE FUNCTION COACHING?

See the Resources at the back of the book for details on and books about the programs mentioned above, along with others.

eight years is a body of clinical trials of new approaches for middle and high school students.

In elementary school three types of school interventions are used. Each requires sufficient teacher training and is more effective with parent engagement. Research and meta-analyses in the past five years have clarified that success depends in part on the quality of the relationships between the teacher and parent and between teacher and child. Your child's principal or a special education teacher may be needed to ensure appropriate skills are in place in the classroom.

1. *Behavioral interventions.* The workhorse of school-based support for kids with ADHD. These interventions require that the teacher use prebehavior prevention (eye contact, cues, prompts, review of rules, activity pacing, teacher movement) and postbehavior consequences (points, computer time, behavior report card) to help children replace an undesirable behavior (calling out in class) with a functionally equivalent and socially acceptable one (raising her hand). Numerous clinical trials and meta-analytic studies support the idea that these approaches help reduce children's disruptive behavior in class and facilitate doing academic work.

2. *Academic interventions* aim to directly teach reading, math, or writing skills. The key elements include incremental teaching of specific skills and can be supplemented by adjunctive techniques like computer-assisted instruction and peer-to-peer instruction; the latter approach most often engages the entire classroom in peer-to-peer tutoring. Although few empirical studies have looked directly at children with ADHD, overall these methods appear promising and provide some benefit to children with emotional and behavioral problems. For children with diagnosable learning disabilities, specific academic training strategies are well supported, such as particular programs for reading disabilities.

3. *Self-regulation interventions.* This is a newer approach that has children identify a self-regulation target behavior (such as attending to an assignment), records their success, and provides feedback or points for success. The conceptual logic is good and single-case trials are promising, but no proper controlled trials have yet been conducted.

Despite numerous educational studies in past decades, little direct study of high school students with ADHD was undertaken until nearly 2010. Now we have evidence, as summarized in a 2014 review in *Child and Adolescent Psychiatric Clinics of North America*, for two new interventions for teens in the school setting. Here, individual interventions have been piloted but have not generated sufficient follow-up to fully evaluate their promise. This is unfortunate as simple interventions might be helpful. The first is note-taking. This intervention involves simply teaching teens with ADHD how to take notes in class effectively. An initial trial over a decade ago showed improvement in their daily assignments but not in quizzes. The second is self-management, building on a large literature that teaches high-schoolers how to manage their schedule and assignments but only recently applied to ADHD. Two very small pilot studies, also a decade ago, were successful in improving homework completion. Neither of these efforts has been followed up. The main energy in the scientific work in the past five to eight years has been in refining and testing more comprehensive efforts at programming in school for teens with ADHD. Two programs have emerged through trials conducted in 2011, 2012, and 2013 and summarized in the 2014 review.

1. *The Challenging Horizons Program (CHP)*. This is a program that combines academic, social, and family skills for the child. While difficult to find and use given its relative newness, the basic program can be carried out as an after-school program by a college student guided by a professional therapist or in a mentoring format in which school personnel meet weekly with students to monitor progress on self-organization skills, test preparation, and study skills. The after-school program is more intensive and is delivered two to three days per week for two hours per session for the entire academic year. Both approaches include periodic parent meetings. The mentoring program, provided during the school day, is more feasible. Randomized trials published from 2011 to 2014 provided empirical support for this program for ADHD, suggesting meaningful reductions in impairment and improvements in academic performance and behavior for participants even in the less intensive mentoring design. Thus, while more confirmation will be helpful, this program, even in the more feasible mentoring format, appears to represent a new and effective option in schools.

2. *The HOPS program (an offshoot of CHP).* HOPS means Homework, Organization, and Planning skills. Here, instead of focusing on social and academic skills, the entire focus is on planning, organization, and time management skills—essentially, executive function coaching in the school context. Thus, this is similar to the organizational skills training discussed earlier, but in this case conducted by the school. Teens are taught a specific system of homework, locker, and desk organization. The intervention is delivered by a school counselor one or two times per week as a short thirty-minute pullout for one semester. Parent meetings are included so that the program can be carried out at home; a reward system is included to maintain teen motivation. The handful of well-designed empirical studies of this approach from 2011 to 2013 reveal consistent improvement in parent-rated, but not teacher-rated, homework and organization skills, mild reduction in ADHD inattention symptoms, and modest improvement in grades. While independent trials are still needed before we can call this a level 1 (definitely efficacious) treatment, it is possibly efficacious and therefore promising.

At this writing these formal programs are not generally available, but it's worth watching for them—we can hope that they will gradually become disseminated, similar to the manual on executive function coaching mentioned earlier.

That said, regardless of the particular in-school support desired, the principal challenge for most parents—and schools—is finding the resources to enable children with ADHD to participate in a strong school-based program. Unless a teacher has special training or supervision or a well-trained classroom aide can be provided, these programs may be out of reach for many schools, which simply don't have the resources for them. Nonetheless, a child with ADHD often will benefit from having a written Individualized Education Program, or IEP, through which some behavioral goals and structure can still be implemented within the resources available to the school. Your behavioral therapist can consult with the school to set up the plan if needed.

The IEP, as some of you already know, is a formal, legal document. In the United States, if you request an IEP in writing, the school must call a meeting to review your child's case and make a determination within ninety days. Some schools adopt an alternative designation called a Section 504 classification. A meeting with school personnel can often produce at least a workable behavioral management plan to help the child get organized and stay on task; parents and teachers generally also benefit from a parent–teacher daily report card, in which the teacher notifies the parent (perhaps via e-mail) of the day's progress, homework, and goals, and the parent follows up with the child at home. Other countries have their own systems.

If you are trying to use a token system (rewards, points, stickers, and so on) to improve your child's frequency of mature behavior or skill learning, or if you are trying to support your child in an organizational coaching approach, a daily report card is a key tool. The teacher can briefly notify you, via e-mail, text, or written note, of key happenings that day relevant to the particular plan you have talked about in advance. This allows you to follow up at home most appropriately and protects your child from falling wildly behind before you are even aware of it. You'll know there is a test tomorrow, or a big assignment due on Friday, or that today was a particularly good or difficult day in the classroom before a negative pattern is established. Most standard parenting programs will include examples of how to use a daily report card, and ready-to-use samples are available in Russell Barkley's ADHD book for parents (see the Resources).

 TAKE-HOME POINTS

Nonmedication Help for Children with ADHD

- Parent counseling/training is well established and effective for managing secondary behavioral ADHD problems, such as defiance, stress level, conflict with others, and outlook.

- ADHD coaching has some promising research data for helping children develop self-regulation and other executive skills often at the center of their ADHD struggles, but mostly for organizing their academic work.

- In both cases, it's important to find a qualified counselor.

- In the United States your child has the right to support from the public

WANT TO READ MORE ABOUT SCHOOL–BASED INTERVENTIONS?

DuPaul, G. J., Gormley, M. J., & Laracy, S. D. (2014). School-based interventions for elementary school students with ADHD. *Child and Adolescent Psychiatric Clinics of North America, 23*(4), 687–697.

Evans, S. W., Langberg, J. M., Egan, T., & Molitor, S. J. (2014). Middle school-based and high school-based interventions for adolescents with ADHD. *Child and Adolescent Psychiatric Clinics of North America, 23*(4), 699–715.

Resources for tracking organizational skills and learning about these types of interventions are available at *www.oucirs.org/resources/educators-mh-professionals.*

Details on the laws that entitle your child to certain accommodations in the public schools are widely available on the Internet. In the United States, search for Individualized Education Program (IEP), Individuals with Disabilities Education Act (IDEA), and Section 504 of the Rehabilitation Act.

> *The school is where your child's ADHD may cause the most distressing problems. Take advantage of the help that the educational system has to offer.*

schools, via two different laws, and many children with ADHD need this assistance.

- Technology-based treatments were reviewed in Chapter 5; recall that computerized cognitive training, while promising, still has insufficient research support to justify your investment at present. Future work may find it helpful in specific learning applications such as math remediation.

MEDICATIONS

Medications are the most well-established and widely used treatment for ADHD. Many available books review the different medications available (see the Resources). I won't repeat that information here but rather point to important recent developments and highlight important but overlooked findings from the research of the past decade or more. I also highlight what you should look for when finding a clinician to work with your child in relation to medication.

The traditional stimulant medications included Ritalin (methylphenidate) and Adderall (an amphetamine salt preparation). These were short-acting preparations given two or three times a day. They "wore off" in a few hours. While numbers varied, the general picture was that over half of children with ADHD would show a positive response to one of these medications, and a significant number of those who didn't would show a positive response to the other, leading to estimates of 70–80 percent "responders." About 20 percent of children with ADHD seemed to fail to respond to either class of medicines. One breakthrough in the past decade or so was the invention of extended- and graduated-release delivery vehicles for these medications, in new packages, such as Concerta, Adderall XR, and Focalin. These reduced side effects, and there is some (less consistent) evidence that children taking them had fewer of the ups and downs of mood or symptoms throughout the day that sometimes resulted from the more frequently administered medication, leading to more consistent improvements in behavior. If you've gone to a doctor for your child's ADHD recently, chances are one of these newer compounds was offered.

Critical Scientific Findings

As noted earlier, the MTA study found that medication plus behavioral treatment was most powerful in eliminating symptoms and also helped the most with associated mood and other problems. But the positive medication effects disappeared sometime after medication was stopped, meaning medication suppresses symptoms but does not cure ADHD. This makes sense. Medications can help children's symptoms quiet down but cannot provide them with the skills and competencies they require to succeed at school or in life. Therefore, skill building is a vital adjunct to medication most of the time.

Hidden in those data was another disturbing finding: the community "controls," the children picked from the general community rather than treated as part of the actual research study, did not do nearly as well. About 70 percent of these kids were being treated with stimulant medication by their doctor, and after fourteen months of treatment, only

25 percent of them experienced total symptom remission, compared to 60 percent in the experimental protocol. This suggests that medication treatment in the community is often delivered poorly.

> ADHD medication treatment often does not meet the standards of practice that help children get the most out of it.

In the study protocol, children's medication dose was shifted systematically over a four-week period, with daily dosage changes and behavioral ratings by parents and teachers. Then the physician saw the family weekly for thirty minutes to continue to adjust the dose as needed, taking into account teacher ratings each time. This is far more intensive than most typical care, even though standards of practice today recommend that different doses be considered regardless of apparent response on the initial dose and consideration given to trying two formulations to find the most effective one. Clinicians too often do not follow these steps, either because they are not aware of the standards, because parents are not willing to go through the steps, or because insurance companies do not want to pay for it. However, this systematic approach complies with the practice parameters of the American Academy of Child and Adolescent Psychiatry (AACAP) and doubles the probability of a successful result for your child's treatment.

What to Look for When Seeking a Prescriber for Medication Treatment

One solution is to consult with an expert, experienced psychiatrist about your child's medication choice and dosing. In the United States and most other countries, medication for ADHD has to be prescribed by a licensed physician (MD), physician's assistant (PA), or nurse practitioner (NP). (In a few locations, where these other prescribers are in short supply, the gap has been filled by a small number of psychologists who have obtained extra training and can also prescribe.) Medication should be approached in the context of a comprehensive plan for the child including home and educational plans, as well as consideration of alternative and complementary treatments as discussed in prior chapters. However, in the United States and many other countries, generalist health care providers just have too many bases to cover and haven't always been able

to develop a high level of expertise in specialized developmental problems. As a result, they sometimes cannot offer all of the following "ideal"
qualifications:

- Expertise and familiarity with all the different ADHD medication
  options.
- Conducts or obtains a thorough evaluation of child psychiatric
  and learning functioning.
- Willingness to explain different medication options to you.
- Follows a protocol and systematically tries more than one dose to
  find the best.
- Has you track and rate symptoms and side effects using a stan-
  dardized rating scale.
- Involves the teacher or urges you to obtain teacher ratings (see
  above).
- Observes your child in addition to talking to you.
- Meets with you frequently until the situation stabilizes.
- Available to coordinate with your behavioral therapist to maxi-
  mize synergy.

I recommend an integrative approach, in which medication is considered in the context of a comprehensive health and development plan
for the child, including home and educational plans, as well as consideration of alternative and complementary approaches to support the child's
functioning, as discussed in Chapters 3–7.

Do All Stimulants Do the Same Thing?

No. The stimulant medications vary in how they physically deliver the
drug to the body, in their effects on brain communication, and in how
patients feel. They vary as well in the ratio of immediate versus delayed
release, in how long until they take effect, and in how long their effect
lasts. So it is important to discuss this in some detail with your physician
to have an accurate expectation of the medication effect. For example,
if you are more concerned about symptom control in the first part of

the day, your physician may select a formulation with a higher ratio of immediate- versus delayed-release medicine. If you are concerned about sleep, this ratio may be reversed. For example, one expert review noted that Concerta may provide twelve hours of "effect"—but at the expense of a weaker effect than another formulation, particularly in the first half of the day. Breadth and depth may have to be traded off, as it were.

Recent evidence from expert systematic reviews attempts to compare the effects of these medications. Practically no studies compare the amphetamines. But several studies have compared the methylphenidate compounds to one another. A handful of meta-analyses have also attempted to compare effects of a given pair of medicines. Perhaps the best summary of this comes from a collaborative expert systematic review published in BMC *Psychiatry* in 2013, which compiled individual "head-to-head" studies as well as prior meta-analyses and reviews. Nearly all the head-to-head comparisons involved Concerta, so it has the advantage and disadvantage of being the most studied. The authors reported the following based on the limited data available in terms of ADHD symptom relief. Based on individual head-to-head comparisons:

- Ritalin LA was superior to Concerta over one to six hours.

- Focalin XR was superior to Concerta over four to six hours but equivalent over eight to ten hours.

- Side effects were similar for all preparations.

- Girls and boys respond differently, with girls tending to respond more quickly and to have effects wear off sooner as the day progresses.

- Individual variation was greater than group differences, so careful individual monitoring remains key. No one medicine is superior for all children.

- Higher doses resulted in a better response on average. (But this is "curvilinear"—that is, at some point the dose gets too high and is actually less effective. So be aware of the risk of overshooting; dosing should still start low and build up.)

- There was some evidence that adults respond better to short-acting than long-acting methylphenidate formulations, although this was disputed.

The study authors offered the following practical recommendations:

- When a partial effect is seen with one methylphenidate formulation, try a second methylphenidate formulation rather than switching right away to an amphetamine formulation.
- Adjust the dose for a satisfactory morning response first.
- Then track the child's response the rest of the day and adjust further if needed.

Finally, individual child response is very complex. Work on the genetic factors that influence metabolism of the drug is very active and over time may yield better ways to personalize the prescribing of medications. Meanwhile, we can't yet predict with confidence which children will respond to a given medication. All we know for sure is that these determinants are complex and that is why it is important to try a child on different dosages and medications. Many other medications, such as Strattera, are not well studied in comparative analyses.

Do Stimulants Harm Brain Growth or Development?

This is a major concern of many parents today. It is a reasonable question because we do know that the brain adapts to drug use by changing its chemical signaling and growth in numerous ways. Data on the specific effects of low-dose stimulant treatment in children that addresses this point are limited. However, what we do have is generally reassuring. Let's walk through this. Two kinds of information inform us here.

Animal Experiments. The first is animal studies. Most studies give various doses of methylphenidate (Ritalin) to rats and measure brain chemicals, then later examine the brain itself. These studies are powerful because they have (1) experimental control and (2) actual examination of the brain under a microscope. These studies therefore provide information about brain changes even at the cellular level. However, they are limited because the animals metabolize the drug differently than humans do. And results are decidedly mixed. Most concerning are several studies that show increased oxidative stress and cell damage in the prefrontal

FAQ: DO STIMULANTS CAUSE TICS?

This is a common parent concern. The FDA requires a warning on stimulant labels saying that they may exacerbate or cause tics. Systematic reviews in the past decade have overturned this conclusion. Here's what seems to be going on. Children with ADHD subsequently develop tic disorder in about 20 percent of cases, even when untreated, because there is a poorly understood and probably genetic relationship between ADHD and tic disorders. (One pathway is simply that serious tic disorders sometimes come on with ADHD symptoms.) Therefore, if a physician starts your child on a stimulant, tics may appear subsequently by chance. Their appearance may have occurred anyway, rather than being caused by the stimulant. The coincidence appears to be a relationship—but it is really only a coincidence. This noncausal correlation was understood by simply looking at rates of tic onset in ADHD with and without stimulant medication—those studies find no difference. The consensus evidence now seems to be that stimulants likely do not increase risk for tics. However, if a child has ADHD with tic disorder, alternative medications can be used effectively, such as guanfacine. It also appears that if in fact a stimulant did trigger tics, the tics typically go away when the stimulant is stopped.

FAQ: DO STIMULANTS STUNT PHYSICAL GROWTH?

This has been one of the most controversial issues in the ADHD literature for decades. The issue arises because stimulants suppress appetite. Contradictory findings abound, and studies continue to emerge annually. A careful summary of the MTA data published in 2015 concluded that treatment caused some growth suppression after ten years of about one inch in final height. However, two new, albeit smaller studies published in 2016 both conclude that stimulant treatments can cause temporary slowdown in rate of growth but did not seem to change the rate of overall physical maturation or final height or bone length. In short, controversy remains about height suppression with sustained stimulant use. It may be that the disagreements disguise substantial individual variation in response to stimulants in relation to growth. Your prescribing physician will carefully track your child's growth at each visit and track whether he is remaining on the same growth curve over time.

WANT TO READ THE LATEST EVIDENCE ON STIMULANTS, TICS, AND PHYSICAL GROWTH?

Bloch, M. H. (2012). Misplaced fear?: FDA contraindication to psychostimulant use in children with tics. *Evidence-Based Child Health, 7*(4), 1231–1234.

Pringsheim, T., & Steeves, T. (2011). Pharmacological treatment for Attention Deficit Hyperactivity Disorder (ADHD) in children with comorbid tic disorders. *Cochrane Database of Systematic Reviews, 4,* CD007990.

Hinshaw, S. P., Arnold, L. E., & MTA Cooperative Group. (2015). Attention-deficit hyperactivity disorder, multimodal treatment, and longitudinal outcome: Evidence, paradox, and challenge. *Wiley Interdisciplinary Reviews: Cognitive Science, 6*(1), 39–52.

Poulton, A. S., Bui, Q., Melzer, E., & Evans, R. (2016). Stimulant medication effects on growth and bone age in children with attention-deficit/hyperactivity disorder: A prospective cohort study. *International Clinical Psychopharmacology, 31*(2), 93–99.

Harstad, E. B., Weaver, A. L., Katusic, S. K., Colligan, R. C., Kumar, S., Chan, E., et al. (2014). ADHD, stimulant treatment, and growth: A longitudinal study. *Pediatrics, 134*(4), e935–e944.

Research is conflicted on whether long-term stimulant use can cause up to a one-inch loss of final height and whether this is only a temporary slowing or a permanent outcome. Make sure the prescribing doctor tracks your child's growth closely.

cortex. The caveat is that dosages in these studies were typically two to ten times more than would be given to human children. While rodents metabolize stimulants differently than humans do (possibly justifying those dosages), this dosage difference still makes it difficult to be sure the studies are reflecting what happens under medical treatment with stimulants in human children. Further, even these brain changes often did not correlate to behavior changes in the animals, at least on measures examined so far. Nonetheless, these results have to give us pause.

It is difficult to generalize from rodents to humans for other reasons too—their brains and behaviors are quite different from ours. Therefore, of particular interest was a study of monkeys published in 2012. Scientists gave the juvenile monkeys a clinical-level dose of methylphenidate

(Concerta) for a year. They confirmed that the blood levels of the drug were exactly what a clinician would see in a human child treated for ADHD. Half of the animals got a placebo. The scientists used a type of brain imaging called PET (positron emission tomography) to observe changes in dopamine receptors in key parts of the brain while the animals were alive (note this requires radioactive isotopes and so is not ethical in human children). Recall that dopamine is one of the most important neurotransmitters involved in ADHD, and it is the brain chemical that Ritalin primarily works on when treating ADHD. Those scientists concluded, reassuringly, that there was no effect of the drug on the development of these dopamine receptors. However, their data analysis had weaknesses that make this conclusion only partly convincing. Also, the number of animals was necessarily few (such studies are very expensive), so the statistical power to detect effects was low. Finally, PET imaging cannot observe the types of oxidative stress seen in the rodent studies. Nonetheless, this study is still somewhat reassuring.

Human Brain Imaging. The second type of study uses brain imaging, such as magnetic resonance imaging, or MRI, to look at human children who have a history of stimulant medication versus those that do not. Some studies use random assignment to look at short-term stimulant effects on the brain. Others look at long-term usage but for ethical reasons cannot use random assignment. All of these studies look at three principal elements: (1) brain growth, such as size of various gray matter structures; (2) brain activity during cognitive tasks; and (3) brain connectivity—the brain's wiring system.

The most recent and comprehensive expert scientific reviews were reported in 2012 and 2014. Both reviews concluded, quite decisively, that short-term effects are, if anything, *positive* in terms of brain metabolism. Essentially, in the short-term stimulant medications appear to "normalize" the activity of key brain regions on cognitive tasks. This is consistent with the short-term effects of medication on cognition and with the idea explained in Chapter 1 that stimulants "wake up" the brain to improve self-regulation.

The studies that look at *longer-term* use are similarly positive for the most part although not as unequivocally. While there are only about a half dozen of these studies, they consistently show a trend toward *nor-*

malization of brain growth as well as of circuit connections in children who have been taking stimulants for a period of time compared to children who did not. The one caveat was that a minority of these studies saw negative effects on long-term *function* of the prefrontal cortex. Most studies, however, saw the opposite: positive normalization of prefrontal cortex functional response to challenge. The reason for this difference in results is not clear and needs to be understood. Nonetheless, the reviewers concluded that based on these studies stimulant medications probably have a normalizing effect on brain growth in children with ADHD, at least on average.

Finally, one unusual study that used PET imaging of dopamine functioning in young adults is notable. A twelve-month course of methylphenidate treatment resulted in changes in dopamine neurochemistry, in the form of increased availability of a chemical called the dopamine transporter. This may explain the drug's action. However, its impact on function is not clear. The authors noted that this response could lead to the medication gradually wearing off or to "rebound" symptoms when medication is discontinued.

Summary. Overall, the evidence here is somewhat mixed but on balance is reassuring. It is clear that chronic stimulant use (a year or more) causes changes in brain growth and development. However, some, perhaps most, of these changes are positive. At the macro level of structural growth and functional wiring of brain connections, the most likely conclusion is that these effects are beneficial and tend toward normalization of brain growth, at least in children with ADHD. However, at the biochemical level, such as cellular health, the picture is less clear. Animal findings of negative effects of stimulant treatment on brain health are concerning. One possibility is that these can be dismissed on the grounds that perhaps the dosages were too high; or perhaps stimulants have positive effects on ADHD but negative effects on healthy brains. Although reassuring, these interpretations are speculative. The balanced possibility may be that long-term treatment effects are a blend of positive brain growth combined with some negatives in brain biochemistry. The absence of known negative effects on behavior or cognition with chronic use suggests that the overall balance of these competing effects is neutral or positive for development. Even the animal studies have shown no long-term loss of cognitive or behavioral function. Nonetheless, it's important to recognize that these are powerful medications and their use has to be justified by clinical need. In particular, they are not appropriate for ordinary performance enhancement purposes.

Putting this all together, in most instances the risks from stimulant medications for ADHD remain reasonable in relation to their potentially profound benefits in helping children adjust and cope. Perhaps the best way to think about this is that you are choosing between two risk paths. One risk is failing to give sufficient treatment to your child with ADHD. With this choice you risk damage to self-esteem, social development, and academic development. The other risk is giving a medication that could have unknown effects on brain devel-

> *Long-term treatment effects may be a blend of positive brain growth with some negatives in brain biochemistry and neutral or positive effects on behavior and cognition.*

opment, although there is no evidence that these effects harm cognitive or behavioral development or long-term outcome; instead they tend to help in these areas. Overall, in the case where stimulants are clinically beneficial, the nod will generally go toward the idea that treating is a better risk than not treating.

 TAKE-HOME POINTS

Professional Help for ADHD

The principal mainline recommendations for ADHD have not changed. While it's possible we'll see new drugs related to epigenetic effects in the future, this still seems somewhat far off. Alternative treatments, such as biofeedback and computerized cognitive training, continue to receive heavy investigation. Most likely they will continue to be secondary or ancillary treatments. Direct brain stimulation may prove more powerful, but the safety of its use in children will take some time to determine. For the most part, the high-tech approaches are still some distance away from being transformative for kids with ADHD. For the near-term future, the major new research directions to watch for in ADHD treatment are in the psychosocial realm. These include, in particular, better methods for teaching children how to improve their planning, organization, and executive functions, either via individual tutoring (an executive function "coach" or "mentor") or through comprehensive in-school programs. Meanwhile, there's hope that fairly simple, targeted interventions such as note-taking skills may make a meaningful difference for some children. If your child's main problem is being disorganized, losing things, and not keeping track—particularly as the child approaches middle and high school—trying these interventions makes sense.

You now have some updates on the few new findings related to executive function coaching. You should also have some idea of what to look for when the time comes to find a pro to lend a hand. Our task now is to weave together the lifestyle and professional resources so you can put together your own plan—this is the focus of Chapter 9.

 AT A GLANCE

Action Steps for Obtaining Professional Help

- If lifestyle changes (see Chapters 3–7) don't help enough to allow your child to lead a happy, healthy life and succeed in school, get a professional assessment. If your child is significantly impaired by ADHD symptoms or your family relationships are deteriorating, it's time to get professional help.

- Whether it's your pediatrician, a therapist, or a psychiatrist, try to find an expert in ADHD who can follow the practice standards issued by the American Academy of Child and Adolescent Psychiatry (AACAP), The American Academy of Pediatrics, the UK's National Institute for Health and Care Excellence (NICE), or the European guidelines promulgated by the European Society for Child and Adolescent Psychiatry. Find someone who uses a reliable parent training program or ADHD coaching approach and will follow practice standards for finding the best medication treatment for your unique child's needs if medication seems indicated by an evaluation.

9

Tying It All Together

In this final chapter we look at some ways different families might use different parts of the information in this book in varying combinations. This is meant to help you think about what combination of insights might be particularly useful for your family. For some families, the most important may be increasing healthy lifestyle with diet, exercise, and sleep. For others, the critical point may be to reduce the level of emotional stress in the family. For yet another, it may be to address toxic chemical exposure. In all cases, it's possible, even probable, that you'll need to combine these personal steps with professional help, for counseling or medication or both. Except for a fortunate few, most lifestyle interventions, like most professional interventions, are not a total cure, but a partial solution. However, the personal steps you take will often make the professional help work better and may enable your child to get by with less professional or medical support than otherwise—in addition to making your family healthier.

Miguel: The Ambiguity of Preschool ADHD

Maria is pregnant with her second child. She and her husband, Carlos, are excited about the new baby but very nervous for two reasons. The first is that their four-year-old son, Miguel, is already so hard to manage that they are worried about him. They think he must have ADHD. But they've been through two evaluations already and been told he's too young and they should wait it out. They've heard, however, that ADHD can really occur and be diagnosed at his age and don't know what to do. The second concern is about the new baby: Will she develop ADHD? What should they do?

As any first-time parent can attest, it's easy to worry a lot when it's your first child. But it makes sense for Maria and Carlos to do what they can to lower their stress, since they are already getting overloaded and are about to face the substantial demands of a new baby. Here, the clinicians might have done better to identify Miguel's problem as ADHD not otherwise specified and begin some parenting management to help him—and as part of that parent counseling include anticipating and planning how Miguel can welcome the new baby and how Maria and Carlos can manage both children. Now the young parents might have to either go back to one of the prior providers and ask for this service or approach yet another provider to get the guidance they want. A family counselor can help with family management concerns without having the diagnosis of ADHD in hand.

With regard to the new baby, Maria and Carlos can work on their own stress level through mindfulness, relaxation techniques, and social support; of course, getting help with Miguel will help a lot. They can also take care to eat well, minimizing processed foods that have additives, with Maria taking the recommended supplements, especially folate and omega-3. Additionally, they can think about any other steps they can take to have a healthy, toxin-free home, such as keeping an eye on cleaning agents they use.

After the baby is born, Maria plans to breastfeed for about five or six months as she did with Miguel, but she might want to breastfeed for a full twelve months in this case, introducing other foods along the way as appropriate. Finally, during those first twelve to twenty-four months of life, both parents can really take full advantage of any available family leave from work (which varies a lot from country to country, state to state, and job to job) to form a positive, secure bond with the new baby while including Miguel. Then, too, they should try to ask friends and relatives for extra support so they continue to feel life is manageable. While they can't implement all these ideas as they make all the other necessary preparations for a new child, they can pick the parts that are manageable for them and get to the others later.

Max: Reversing the Academic Spiral to Prepare for High School

At thirteen Max had barely finished eighth grade. His problems with concentrating, losing his assignments, lacking motivation, and being restless and spaced out in class had worsened each year, culminating in near failure in junior high. His parents, Corinne and David, had real concerns about his ability to manage freshman year in high school. They had long wondered if Max had ADHD, and now they suspected he might have depression as well, because Corinne had struggled off and on with depression for much of her life. To make matters worse, Max was playing video games in his room all evening every evening. When David or Corinne attempted to restrict his gaming, Max overreacted, leading to nasty arguments and blowups.

After some reflection and discussion, David and Corinne decided to push Max to enroll in the city's summer youth basketball league. Adult and college-age volunteers were organizing hour-long pickup games every afternoon and setting up teams for a tournament later in the summer. At first they thought basketball would at least get Max out of the house, but they had heard it might help his attention and mood too. Once Max was playing he enjoyed it; he was a decent player, the players were competitive, and play was fast-paced and well supervised. Max was running and breathing hard much of the time. But he needed frequent cajoling to get out the door.

The situation got easier after his parents worked out a compromise with Max: he could play video games for one hour each night if he maintained attendance at the basketball camp, so long as he quit and went to bed by 10:00 P.M. At the same time, after reading an article about sleep problems, they moved his computer out of his room and into the family room. Max was anything but thrilled, complaining that he needed privacy to joke with his friends online during the game. But he relented when his parents agreed not to eavesdrop and assured him they had their own stuff to do. He reluctantly agreed that he needed to sleep better anyway.

Meanwhile, the daily exercise gradually seemed to revive Max. He was calmer, more confident, and more relaxed about how much video game time he got. Noticing this, in the fall his parents pushed him again.

They discussed with him the importance of exercise and regular sleep to his health and academics. Max didn't seem that interested in this concept, but he accepted a new agreement that during freshman year he could again play video games an hour each evening on two conditions: he either played basketball or ran three miles daily after school, turned in at least 90 percent of his homework on time, and maintained a B average. The running alternative worked out because some of the kids on the freshman team were running with the cross-country team during their practice to get in shape. Again, Corinne and David required Max to quit the computer and go to bed by 10:00 P.M. The sleep article had mentioned blue light from screens affecting sleep, so they invested in an orange filter for the computer monitor. All this took some negotiating, and in the end Max's parents had to throw in a deal sweetener—driver's education class could start next summer if he maintained this agreement all year. After a few weeks, Max got his new habits going.

It still wasn't a bed of roses. Corinne had to e-mail Max's teachers regularly to track his homework and make sure he hit the 90 percent mark. David had to visit basketball or cross-country practices at least once a week to encourage Max when Max felt like skipping or quitting. And David met with the coach a couple of times to explain their effort to use exercise to help Max keep his grades up so the coach could make sure Max was on the court enough to get in plenty of running. David made sure the coach knew he wasn't trying to get Max more playing time in the games—just making sure he got plenty of exercise. Fortunately, the ninth-grade coach shared their priorities; he was doubling as a science teacher and wanted the kids to be healthy and get good grades. David and Corinne had to carve out some time each week to make sure they sat down and talked and coordinated with each other as well.

By October, Max was able to sit and do his homework in the evening and could handle parental limits on the videogames without getting too wound up about it. The overreactions had stopped. He was still pretty disorganized, but now he was motivated and at least sitting and taking notes in class, and he wasn't so restless. To further help him handle the more complicated high school schedule, Corinne found a reputable executive function coach. Ms. Davidson had a master's degree in special education and had decided to start her own executive function coaching and tutoring business. She enjoyed teenagers and offered Max both online and in-person options for learning the teenagers' organizing system she liked. Max chose the online option, where he and Ms. Davidson could chat in real time while he learned how to organize his planner, his books, and his checklists for school. She spent eight weekly sessions online with Max, showing him how to organize his books, schedule, and homework. These types of interventions easily fall apart afterward as kids and parents forget the course contents, so in this case Ms. Davidson invited Max and his parents to three booster sessions scheduled once a month. This helped Max keep using the parts of the program that worked for him.

David, who enjoyed systems, learned the system too so he could help Max implement it. The system enabled Max to track his own homework and prove he was hitting his 90 percent completion mark, so Corinne could e-mail less often with the teachers. Max was able to maintain the B average, and he didn't seem to need further help for ADHD or depression.

In this case, a few additional details are interesting. Corinne had a history of depression stemming from her own traumatic youth. It may be that she carried a genetic predisposition that Max had inherited, or it may be that Corinne carried epigenetic changes associated with her own adversities, which Max had inherited. The steady exercise may have helped reverse those prior epigenetic marks, as research studies in animals have shown can happen. Sleep problems may have complicated both mood and attention; the combination of exercise and reasonable (if generous) limits on screen time likely helped sleep, creating a virtuous cycle. Corinne and David had to create a behavioral plan that they negotiated with Max and create specific targets for him to change his habits. They also had to carve out a little extra time and coordinate with the school to make things work. But once Max had settled down emotionally and was less restless and able to pay attention, the problem was narrowed to just being disorganized. Then the executive function coach was able to take him the rest of the way toward success with some organizational skills training, booster sessions, and in this case active parent engagement in the process.

Max probably had ADHD, perhaps combined with a mild mood disorder, although he was never formally diagnosed. If so, the form of dysregulation he experienced revealed itself as low activation and poor mental control. He wasn't terribly hyperactive, and he wasn't particularly in a sad mood, but he was irritable, spoke impulsively, and had very poor attention. In this case, his self-regulation problems were brought back on track with minimal outside help and lots of at-home changes.

Latonya: Food for the Mind and Mood

Nine-year-old Latonya was inattentive, disorganized, very impulsive (blurting out in class), hyperactive, always on the go, and unhappy. She frequently broke down crying during dinner or had a tantrum over some small chore. She seemed very intelligent, but she could not get her homework done or keep up with school. She frequently complained of headaches or stomachaches, seemingly to get out of going to school. Her mother, Charisse, was a hospital receptionist. She and Latonya's father, Andre, had divorced when Latonya was three. Latonya visited Andre on Wednesday evenings and every other weekend. Charisse had tried behavior plans and felt they did not work. Latonya's pediatrician had diagnosed her with ADHD a year ago. She was taking Concerta, but it seemed to have only a partial effect on her restlessness, poor attention, disorganization, and unhappiness. Charisse felt that while the Concerta helped only partially, without it things were even worse. But with it, things were still not sustainable.

Latonya seemed to get to bed and sleep just fine; she had nightmares from time to time but seemed rested and alert in the morning. Charisse had tried enrolling Latonya in a dance class for exercise. Latonya enjoyed it, but there was no real change in her attention or behavior. She was still having meltdowns practically every day and was irritable, restless, and out of her seat at school, and she had a negative attitude most of the time at home. Charisse was reading about healthy foods and wondered about diet. She had a friend who was very interested in diet who suggested removing the most allergenic foods and substituting other foods.

Charisse therefore made gradual changes over a six-week period. She found some fish oil supplements and started giving these to Latonya and taking them herself. She started mixing cow's milk with coconut milk in a gradually increasing ratio. Latonya got used to it and was fine with the coconut milk after a couple of weeks. Charisse replaced their bread with wheat-free bread; after trying a few flavorless brands she was able to locate a tasty brand available at a nearby health food store. Checking with her knowledgeable friend, she also started checking labels to avoid soy products, quit offering nuts as a snack, and began reading labels to avoid food additives and processed food. She had to find a new grocery store that had a better selection of healthy, tasty food. After that Charisse was able to buy the food she wanted, although she winced at the extra cost. The most difficult problem was that Latonya really loved her sugary red sippy juice. Charisse had to gradually substitute pure apple juice without added sugar. She motivated Latonya with a promise of a glass of chocolate coconut milk on the weekends. While not ideal, that little bit of sugar, with no other color additives, was okay.

Andre was not very interested in these efforts, but he agreed to help with getting rid of the red juice, and he agreed to serve Latonya the wheat-free bread and coconut milk if Charisse would provide it. Charisse resented that he would not do more but after thinking it over decided it wasn't much trouble. So Charisse brought these foods along when she dropped Latonya off every other weekend, and Andre followed through and served these foods to Latonya.

After about eight weeks, the new diet was in place, and after about ten weeks Charisse noticed some real changes were occurring. Latonya was not nearly so restless or hyperactive; she was also less irritable and had gone two weeks without a tantrum. She seemed to be in a better mood and had a better attitude. She also seemed able to remember instructions; instead of complaining when given an instruction, she complied. She was still inattentive at school but not nearly as much as before. Now that she was staying in her seat, the teacher felt the attention problems were quite manageable. By four months later, a new normal seemed to be in place. The new diet and supplements had helped, and although she was still taking Concerta, Latonya was now managing to get Bs and even one A in school. Life at home was far more pleasant. Charisse now found that the positive parenting strategies she had tried to use from the books she bought were actually working, whereas before they hadn't seemed to do any good.

In Latonya's case, there seemed to be an undetected food sensitivity that was driving an irritable mood and contributing to her inattention. In retrospect, her stomachaches and headaches may have provided a clue to that problem, although those symptoms may be absent even when there is a food sensitivity. Latonya's ADHD, or dysregulation problem, included a marked restlessness and hyperactivity—motor symptoms—while her attention problems were mild when her restlessness settled down. She had a negative mood, but in retrospect this may have been due to not feeling well rather than only to poor self-regulation. The food sensitivity may explain why the medication worked only partly and why efforts at positive parenting or behavior management, as well as exercise, weren't succeeding. The sensitivity may have been due to Latonya having a certain genotype that caused extra inflammation when she ate these foods or food additives. To overcome that genetic risk, she needed a different environment. Once again, we see that parental effort to motivate the child was an important part of the puzzle, and cooperating with other adults, in this case Latonya's father, helped make things work. Charisse benefited from having a knowledgeable friend. But without that, she might have obtained a nutritionist referral from her pediatrician to get the same results.

Nicholas: Keeping Things Calm So He Can Carry On

At age seven, Nicholas already seemed to have serious problems. At home and at school he was erupting into tantrums that lasted for an hour or more almost daily and flunking his classes. His mother, Diane, was a former nurse who had opted to be a full-time mom to manage both his problems and the challenge of caring for his three-year-old sister, who had Down syndrome. His father, Bill, was self-employed in a one-man plumbing business shop; but with money tight due to medical bills and credit card payments, he was taking on a lot of extra hours, up to twelve hours a day and weekends. He was thinking of hiring an assistant to reduce his workload but not sure the numbers would add up. Bill and Diane were arguing frequently; between Nick's tantrums, the baby's needs, and stress over money, the home was anything but a haven. Nick's tantrums were so severe that the doctor had diagnosed both ADHD and a disruptive mood disorder and put Nick on two different psychiatric medications—Concerta and Prozac, which only partially controlled the problem. The pediatrician mentioned that exercise or diet might help Nick, but Diane didn't have the mental energy to even think about it.

Meanwhile, Bill couldn't stand the knot that formed in his stomach when he heard the kids crying endlessly or when he argued with Diane, who complained that he didn't help out enough with the kids, while he countered that she didn't understand their financial predicament or why he had to work so much. Most evenings Bill retreated to the basement family room to zone out with TV and a beer. Then one night, in the midst of meltdowns all around, the two parents had had enough. They looked at each other, called Bill's sister to watch the kids, and went out for a heart-to-heart talk. They agreed they had to create a better tone at home. Money worries were eating at Bill, and Diane was overwhelmed. They realized they were committed to each other and the family, but that they needed some help. They made some decisions. Diane agreed to stop discussing Bill's work hours until they could see a counselor, while in return Bill agreed to turn off the TV, put away the beer, and help with bedtimes.

The next day, Bill met with a financial counselor at the bank, who helped the family refinance some debt and come up with a business plan for his company that involved part-time help for now and growth of the business, and made shorter working hours possible for Bill. Now he got home for dinner every night, and he and Diane took turns getting the kids to bed. Diane and Bill also saw a marriage counselor several times, who helped them learn basic communication, teamwork, and relaxation strategies and also helped them talk and connect about the grief both had felt, but never really shared, that their cherished second child had Down syndrome.

After three months, they realized that Nick's tantrums were now happening only once a week instead of daily, and that if they just sent Nick to his room to calm down, he was back out and ready to play in thirty minutes instead of going on all evening. Their daughter seemed happier too. Eventually, Nick was able to be tapered off the Prozac and shifted to a reduced dose of Concerta. Most days at school were good ones, and he maintained grade-level learning.

Exercise or nutrition changes were beyond reach for this family, at least initially, and they may not have helped anyway. Financial challenges, grief, and other stressors had overwhelmed both parents emotionally, and Nick had been melting down partially in response to this context. While a resilient child might manage even when parents are going through these all-too-common hardships, Nick could not. It turned out that Nick was quite stress sensitive. He may have picked this up as an epigenetically influenced tendency from Diane's stressful pregnancy with him, when she got laid off from work. Both Bill and Diane may have been prone to losing their tempers, perhaps from either genetic tendencies or their own earlier learning in their families of origin. Yet the stresses they faced were all too real. Fortunately, Diane and Bill were willing to make some changes before it was too late. They saved Nick by saving themselves. They recommitted, got the counseling help they needed, and turned things around. Although Nick did meet the criteria for ADHD, his was one of those cases in which self-regulation problems were made a lot worse due to his sensitivity to emotional input and a limited capacity to adjust to emotional intensity in this overwhelmed household. He was inattentive but also had emotional regulation challenges. Remember, kids with ADHD often are more responsive to environmental stressors precisely because they don't regulate well. In this case, the spiral that he and his parents were caught up in was interrupted, and Nick settled into a better zone.

Jessica and Rachel: Different Pictures of ADHD

The children just described illustrate that different combinations of treatments work for different individuals. I chose to tell stories that showed a link between the form of the problem and why the intervention worked, but that won't typically be very clear in real life. Because self-regulation is a complex capacity with various components (see Chapter 1), ADHD can manifest in different ways at different times and with different co-occurring problems. This fact can not only obscure a link between the form of a problem and an effective intervention but also create even more complications when the genetic predisposition toward ADHD surfaces in more than one child in a family.

Sisters Jessica, eleven, and Rachel, ten, each had a type of ADHD, but because they had such different personalities, the problems they struggled with were quite distinct. Rachel was uncoordinated and gangly and had terrible handwriting. Her temperament was irritable. When things went wrong she had a tantrum that was difficult to contain, and she was often in a bad mood, although this problem was most noticeable at home. Rachel was withdrawn at school. She struggled to learn to read, and the school decided in third grade that she had a learning disability and needed special education. She was also diagnosed with ADHD around that time. Her single mom, a nurse, was reluctant to try stimulant medication. So instead, her mother concentrated on trying to find the right school environment and getting her extra support. She also had to work with the tantrums, which was an ongoing struggle. She liked to sing, and as she got older she wanted to get more serious about music. Rachel needed help with attention and organization, help with focus, and help coping with disappointment.

Jessica presented a different picture. Smart and athletic, she was able to form a group of friends. Yet she was extremely impulsive, grabbing other kids' things, blurting out disruptive comments in class, and getting in a loud argument and making a big scene if another child accidentally bumped into her. She had an exuberant style, was often in a good mood, easily got angry but quickly settled down, and loved a challenge. She loved to play soccer, loved competition, and needed a lot of physical activity during the day to be able to settle down in the evening. If she didn't get to ride her bike for an hour, play soccer for a while, or take a long walk with her mother, she was very hard to manage in the evening. She was diagnosed with ADHD, also in third grade. Her mother accepted a recommendation for some behavioral programs to help Jessica get better control of her behavioral problems, contain her outbursts and scenes at school, and get enough activity. It was clear that Jessica needed both plenty of exercise and real structure to make it.

It's common for siblings to be surprisingly different from one another, even though they grow up in the same family. Here both girls had ADHD, but it manifested differently. Rachel was relatively introverted, had a tendency toward negative feelings, and had coordination and learning problems; her social and emotional development were very different than her sister's. Jessica was blessed with social and physical gifts but had an exuberant impulsivity and thus a different form of poor self-regulation. Each needed a distinct approach. While both girls may have benefited from stimulant medication, in this case the parent wanted to try without medication and was able to make changes in the children's environment to get them on track.

TAKE-HOME POINTS

Putting It All Together

ADHD results from a complex interplay of child biology, partly rooted in genes and partly in epigenetic effects, and environmental context. ADHD is not caused by one single factor, like excessive use of video games or "bad" genes. Epigenetics has shown us that the environmental aspects play a bigger role than previously thought, operating in tandem with genetic liability. This is what each of these families was able to use to its advantage. By changing some aspects of the complex mix affecting the child, they were able to help the child get back on course.

What works for a child won't necessarily pay off right away. But in each case above, once the family found the right mix, the situation began to turn around within weeks or months. While there are no guarantees, *this really does happen, and it can happen for you.*

Professional support and personal lifestyle changes can nicely augment each other. For the families described here, I didn't emphasize the professional help much, but it's important to balance the realization that your child's environment can make a real difference in success with acceptance of the need for some professional help as well—at some point, in some way, in most cases. In fact, the combination of the two will be the most common picture in a successful turnaround for children with ADHD. Lifestyle changes are likely to help, and to amplify the benefit of professional help or to reduce the amount of it you need, but they won't be a panacea.

The principles we are talking about apply whether or not a child formally meets criteria for ADHD. ADHD is probably the extreme end of a dimension of behavior and self-regulation in many instances. Wherever a child is on that continuum, if she is being impaired by these problems, then the research summarized in this book may be relevant. If your efforts to manage the problems on your own aren't working, get a professional evaluation. Use the guidelines for what to look for in Chapter 8. Whether or not your child gets a diagnosis of ADHD, the evaluation can help clarify the nature of the problem, and the pro can help you fine-tune how you implement your strategy. Whether it is behavioral management, diet, stress reduction, or, for that matter, medications, the intervention can range from ineffective to very effective depending in part on how carefully it is implemented. Getting the right pro in your corner can help you make sure you hit all the right notes.

The dynamics I described in the families profiled in this chapter can happen in conjunction with almost any cultural context. I have seen pictures like those described in observant Christian, Muslim, and Jewish homes as well as in secular or nonreligious homes, and in families that are white, African American, Hispanic/Latino, Asian American, and of mixed race. I work in the United States, but my colleagues in many other countries write and talk about very recognizable situations when we meet at conferences. In each of these cultural and social contexts, there are of course additional complexities to consider that make your situation unique and specific.

Changes to your family's routines and decisions about treatment for your child should always be based on what makes the most sense for your child, you, and your family. Take a look at your own situation. You may feel like you have already tried diet, exercise, medication, and time-outs to no avail. Or you've tried professional help but not the lifestyle changes suggested in this book. Maybe you've taken measures to improve your child's sleep hygiene, including minimizing screen time before bed, but not thought much about exercise or nutrition. The checklist that follows will give you a chance to think through your options— based on what you intuitively think might work best for your child but also on what you can realistically manage. Dietary changes may seem like a huge chore (or simply impractical) for you, while exercise could easily be woven into your lives—that's just one example among many. See where the checklist leads you, try out your top choices, and then always be willing to revise and try something different after giving your first choices a reasonable test period.

You can start this checklist with whichever item seems most easy or accessible to you. In each case, if the first answer doesn't lead you to an immediate next step, move on to the next item.

A Decision Tree for Where to Start

Is the problem feeling like an emergency, like there's no space to work it through?

- Yes → Get professional consultation now and add lifestyle changes as you go.
  - See Chapter 8 for more on professional help. See Chapters 3–7 for lifestyle changes.

- Yes, but this is mainly due to conflict at home, not school. Start with behavioral counseling, adding other lifestyle changes as you go.
  - See Chapter 8.

- Yes, and your child is "out of control" everywhere. You may need to start with medication, then you can try to back it off as other supports come online.
  - See Chapter 8 for more on medication.

- No → Consider some lifestyle changes and see how far you get, then get professional help once you hit the limits.
  - See Chapters 3–7 first, then Chapter 8.

To help you choose where to start, code each action step that follows for how relevant and how easy it will be to take, using the suggested codes below.

Code *relevance* like this:

A. Yes, this strikes me as a likely part of the puzzle and seems important.

B. Maybe, but I'm not sure this is the main thing we need to do.

C. No, we already do this/I'm sure this area is fine.

Code *ease of implementation* like this:

A. Yes—I can do this starting this week. I'll make the first move on it today.

B. Maybe—I'd have to build up some energy, but I can make this happen with some effort.

C. No—this is beyond me right now.

Action step	Relevance	Ease of implementation
Increase child's exercise to sixty minutes of moderate/vigorous daily (see Chapter 4; see action steps on pages 97–98)	____	____

Possibilities:

- Can the child join in on your exercise routine?
- Can you two start a fitness routine together?
- Can your child join a sports team (if suitable; see pages 90–92)?
- Can your child get involved in a vigorous nonteam activity (for example, hiking, cycling, running, rock climbing, dance)?
- Can you make desirable sedentary activities (such as video games) contingent on meeting daily exercise goals?
- Can you build in times for exercise before school (may depend on changing sleep schedule)?
- Can your child be directed to active outdoor play with siblings or peers on a more regular basis?

| Add daily omega-3 supplement or regular (at least three times per week) intake of coldwater fish (see Chapter 3; see action steps on pages 85–87) | ____ | ____ |

Possibilities:

- Can you identify a reputable health food/vitamin store or online seller?
- Can you introduce salmon, sardines, or mackerel into your family's diet?
- Can you add walnuts, flaxseeds, or chia seeds to salads or other dishes?

Action step	Relevance	Ease of implementation
Eliminate food coloring and preservatives by buying only fresh food and food with ingredients I recognize and could use at home (see Chapter 3; see action steps on pages 85–87)	____	____

Possibilities:

- Can you buy only organic produce?
- Can you switch to a higher percentage of organic foods while staying on budget?
- If organic food is prohibitively expensive, can you focus on whole, natural foods (fresh fruits, vegetables, meat, fish, and grains versus boxed, bagged, or frozen products)?
- Can you grow your own vegetables or join a co-op?
- Can you shop at farmers' markets?
- Can you shop the outer aisles of supermarkets?
- Can you avoid packaged or processed food?
- Can you cut out or cut down on refined sugar in foods by eliminating soft drinks, juices, sweets, and processed carbs except on special occasions?

Action step	Relevance	Ease of implementation
Eliminate commercial cleaning and pest-control products and substitute EPA-approved products when necessary (see Chapter 6; see action steps on pages 159–160)	____	____

Possibilities:

- Can you repair and repaint any household surface painted before 1980?
- Can you use natural cleaning substances like vinegar, lemon juice, and baking soda instead of chemical-filled commercial products?
- Can you avoid pesticides in your house and yard (except natural substances like boric acid)?
- Can you look for the EPA label on household products to reduce toxic ingredients? (See the Resources at the back of this book.)
- Can you switch from canned to frozen or fresh vegetables and fruits?
- Can you purchase your baby's toys through a nontoxic manufacturer? (See the Resources on at back of this book.)
- Can you breastfeed your baby for twelve to twenty-four months to help protect them from toxicant exposures and other early stressors?

Action step	Relevance	Ease of implementation

- Can you take action to reduce your own and your family's stress (see Chapter 7) to counteract the effects of exposure to pollutants?
- Can you use a high-quality, properly certified water filter in your house? (See the Resources.)

Get a handle on parent/child/family stress
by changing schedules, using meditation or
relaxation strategies, exercise, social support,
or parent counseling (see Chapter 7; see
action steps on pages 181–182)   ____   ____

Possibilities:

- Can you see a counselor or get help with obligations if under excess stress?
- Can you learn—and teach your child—relaxation techniques? (See the Resources.)
- Can you provide the supports your child needs to boost resilience to stress (see pages 185–188)?

Improve child sleep routine or sleep amount
with a fresh bedtime schedule that's
enjoyable and feasible (see Chapter 4; see
action steps on pages 110–111)   ____   ____

Possibilities:

- Can you establish a consistent bedtime to allow your child sufficient sleep for his or her age (see the table on page 104)?
- Can you eliminate use of screens for an hour before bed?
- Can you remove any TVs or other screens from your child's bedroom?
- Can you create a relaxing, enjoyable bedtime routine?
- Can you ensure that stimulant use doesn't interfere with your child's sleep?
- Can you add incentives for getting to bed on time?

Reduce blue screen exposure and screen
media time, especially the hour before
bedtime (see Chapters 4 and 5; see the FAQ
on page 124)   ____   ____

Possibilities:

- Can you limit screen media use to a certain maximum amount of time per day?
- Can you substitute something positive (exercise?) for shortened screen time?
- Can you put an orange filter on your child's computer?
- Can you keep tablets and smartphones away from the table at family mealtimes?
- Can you make screen time an earned privilege instead of an entitlement?

Working with Professionals

In Chapter 8 we reviewed what the science tells us about the various types of professional help for children with ADHD and their families. I listed the qualifications you should seek to ensure that you will get qualified help and described the circumstances that might call for particular types of help in diagnosis and treatment. But professional treatment is, of course, a two-way street. Even when you find professionals that you like and trust, you will have to feel comfortable establishing a balance between following their recommendations and making your own questions and concerns known. Professionals appreciate it when a client has done some homework, has some ideas, and is motivated. At the same time, if you aren't going to follow their advice, most professionals will wonder why you even called them in the first place. So you should be open to the professionals' recommendations, but a good professional also will listen to your ideas. Ideally, a meeting of the minds will take place. Good clinicians will be comfortable explaining why a particular idea isn't suitable in your child's case or, quite often, will help you try your idea in a safe and supported way.

For example, when Hector took his daughter Sonia for an ADHD evaluation, the nurse practitioner recommended a trial of Adderall. It was only after Hector did a little reading and pointed out that Sonia struggled to wake up every morning that the pediatrician took a closer look at her sleep patterns. Then he identified a sleep–wake phase disorder. Given the very short time available for the medical consultation, the physician had simply missed this important clue while focused on ruling out more serious possible disorders such as a thyroid problem or another psychiatric problem. A revised treatment plan involved consult-ing a behavioral counselor to create a new sleep pattern for managing the sleep disorder. Once that was resolved, it was possible to delay the stimulant treatment for a while to see how Sonia would do.

As another example, Doug and Melanie obtained an evaluation for their twelve-year-old son Jerry because of significant ADHD symptoms. ADHD was duly diagnosed and a medication was started. They were given a prescription and told to come back in six months. But after one week on the prescription, they could see that while Jerry was far better during the school day, he was markedly worse in the evening. Every eve-ning he was in one long severe tantrum—a new behavior that was not present before. They did not know what to do—school was improved, but home life was falling apart. They sought a second opinion from a psychiatrist, and after suffering another three weeks of uncertainty got in to see one. The psychiatrist determined that the dosage was too high and causing evening rebound effects. She saw Jerry for three consecutive weeks, adjusting the dose until he had a positive school response and no evening rebound problems. In this case the family changed doctors, but it might have worked as well to take the problem right back to the original prescriber for adjustment.

QUESTIONS TO ASK THE PROFESSIONALS

Here's a short list of questions you can productively ask any clinician you're considering for diagnosis and treatment of your child. You won't necessarily ask every single question, but rather you can draw on those suggested questions that are relevant to your situation. Your goal isn't to come in "guns blazing," but rather to be an active partner in the process and let your clinician know you want to learn and understand. These questions can both help you feel comfortable with your professionals and also help both you and them avoid mistakes. A good professional will appreciate that and be glad you are so engaged. He won't run every test you suggest (nor should he, if it's not needed), but he should have a well-thought-out answer to these questions and appreciate the chance to clar-ify his thinking. Some of these questions may be answered in advance on the clinician's web page or other marketing materials.

Professional Background

- "What is your degree in?"
- "Are you fully licensed in this state?"
- "How long have you been doing this work?"
- "What types of cases or problems do you consider to be your strong suit?"
- "Do you specialize in children?"
- "Do you specialize in behavior problems/ADHD/mental health issues?"
- "What do you need from me to enable you to be maximally helpful to me?"

Diagnostics

- "Are you confident this is not a sleep disorder? What else can I watch for?"
- "Are you confident there is no problem with a zinc, iron, or other nutritional deficiency?"
- "Are you confident this is not a thyroid or other metabolic problem?"
- "We live in an old house/go to an old school/live near an airport: Should we check her blood lead level?"
- "He really doesn't like school/can't read/can't write/doesn't seem to understand math. How can we make sure it's not a learning disability?"
- "His tantrums seem unrelated to events. How do we know it's not depression?"
- "What are the reasons you think this is ADHD? What should I be watching for that would indicate we need a fresh review of diagnostics?"
- "I've heard some kids with ADHD are just low energy and can't get activated. It is possible she has that kind of ADHD rather than depression?"

- "He has a lot of tantrums, but he also has problems getting organized. I've heard these can be connected. Is it possible this is all related to ADHD?"

Treatments

Alternative Treatments

- "Can we try omega-3 supplements?"
- "Can you refer me to a dietician so I can try some healthier foods?"
- "Is it safe for my child to start some more vigorous exercise?"
- "Can you help me get a guideline for establishing a bedtime routine?"

Medication

- "Are you following any particular algorithm in selecting medications?"
- "Is this dose a high dose, low dose, or medium dose?"
- "Why don't we try a different dose of the medication before we change medicines?"
- "Shouldn't we get the teacher to do some brief ratings without knowing whether my child is on medication or not?"
- "Some things are better but some things are worse; can we try a different dose or different medication?"
- "Can I have a list of side effects to watch for?"

Counseling

- "Do you provide parent behavioral counseling?"
- "What does that consist of?"
- "Will you give me specific skills I can try at home or in the office to make sure they work?"
- "Do you follow a certain model or curriculum when you teach parenting skills?"

- "How many meetings will we plan on?"
- "How will we evaluate our progress?"

Self-Care

- "I've been preoccupied by my own problems/mood/conflicts in marriage or at work/health problems/other. Do you think addressing that would help my child? Do you think it is feasible? Can you give me an appropriate referral?"

What's Ahead for Your Child?

Perhaps the most pressing concern for all parents whose child has any kind of problem related to ADHD, self-regulation, or other developmental issues is "What does the future hold?" I have seen many children come to a positive outcome, including several of the children on whom the composite, disguised cases in this book are based. I have already mentioned several resilience factors for children. But in the end, we come back to the big-picture priorities for you as a parent. The non-negotiables are the same whether your child is thriving or struggling. The children who do well invariably had parents who were able to do the following:

1. Convinced their children they cared about them, showed them affection, and, at least some of the time, created positive relationship-building experiences with them year after year.
2. Stayed engaged with their kids—through thick or thin. Never disconnected, gave up, or lost interest. These children knew that no matter what else anybody could say, and no matter how many mistakes they might make, their parents were in it for the long haul with them.
3. Worked on their own issues. These parents tried to work out their own depression, alcohol abuse, past trauma, stress, and marital conflicts by reading self-help books, seeing a counselor, talking to friends, or engaging in self-examination. As a result,

even while they may have felt they were making the same mistakes year after year, they were aware of their own actions, able to hear the perspective of their children, and able to adapt when possible.

4. Established limits of some kind. They may have had limits that were too strict, or not strict enough, but they had rules and tried to hold their kids accountable for following them, confronting them when they broke the rules. These limits weren't always ideal, but they did require the child to deal with rules and limits.

5. Avoided having a consistently harsh/negative style. If they found themselves criticizing their kids too much, they apologized or balanced it out with encouragement. They avoided harsh physical punishment and tried to explain their rules to their children.

This doesn't mean that their relationship with their kids who had ADHD was perfect, that there weren't scars, or real heartbreaks. But the kids made it—they found jobs, made friends, raised families, and forged their own path in life. It also doesn't mean that parents who fall short in some of the areas above can't also get their kids to a positive outcome—but hitting these five targets markedly raises the odds.

I can't overemphasize the importance of self-care. Stress (Chapter 7) is perhaps the most underappreciated influence on environmentally sensitive kids with ADHD. When a parent is overly stressed, it's very difficult for a child to be calm, confident, and learning. Our kids are too dialed in to our state of mind—even when we don't think they are. It makes sense: evolution has taught children that their survival depends on the danger and safety signals from their adult caregivers. Their instincts are wired to monitor us. Furthermore, caring for a child with ADHD is *hard*. It's challenging, draining, demanding, and exhausting. Without an occasional break, your own exercise and sleep, a supportive friend or peer group for yourself, and some good times in your own life, it is very difficult to sustain the journey that your child needs from you. Take care of yourself, and take care of your child. Many of the changes in lifestyle discussed here will help you as well as your child and can be done together as a family.

Where Is the Science Headed?

While the fundamental insight of our era for children's neurodevelopment is the epigenetic paradigm, there is another insight, now capturing
the field of medicine: that body and brain, brain and mind, and body and
mind are connected. The physical and mental health needs of each of us,
and children in particular, are connected. The interplay between us and
our environment and experiences affects both as well. New and exciting
research directions are building on these new, fundamental principles.
A steady stream of papers is starting to map how specific genotypes and
specific environments interact in development. Forthcoming research is
beginning to better map how genes and early experiences are related
to specific aspects of the multifaceted symphony of early brain development. The potential improvements in combined behavioral, lifestyle,
and medical treatments for ADHD are just beginning to be explored.
How the mind responds to different social signals during development
will open new avenues for guiding parents and teachers. In the longer
term, the potential to prevent ADHD entirely is imaginable. We are in a
position to begin to understand the epigenetics of development in coming decades. Recognizing that ADHD is not simply genetic, but arises
through the interaction of genetic liability and experience, should open
new avenues for aggressive study of the limits and possibilities of early
and subsequent environmental interventions, perhaps informed by genotype to target the right approach to the right child.

Recent worldwide surveys funded by the Gates Foundation revealed
in 2013 that neurodevelopmental, mental, and addictive disorders are
the number one cause of morbidity (defined formally as years lived with
disease or disability, but for our purposes is a cumulative loss of quality
of life over the lifetime) in the world compared to any other disease category. This is because they emerge in childhood, during the long period
of brain development. ADHD is one of the major tips of this iceberg
because it emerges early and, unchecked, can lead to numerous associated problems. The problem therefore is serious and requires far more
public investment. At the same time, progress to date is impressive and
exciting. The energy in the scientific community is high, and the future
is bright for new treatments and discoveries. Most nations, including the

United States, don't come close to funding research on these conditions that is proportionate to their health impact—we do a better job funding research on what kills us when we are old after a full life than on what can rob kids of their future when they are young. That may change. Meanwhile, scientific progress in this area is exciting and holds real promise of breakthrough changes to come.

There is ample reason for optimism and hope in your own life too. ADHD tends to be persistent and difficult to change, but change is not impossible. The rough edges can be softened and the hidden gifts made more apparent. Kids can find the niche that works for them. There's often a way to capitalize on the new science that shows us that just as the brain rewires itself with learning, so the genome resets its own volume based on past and recent experience to ensure that we continue to grow and adapt. We are learning, slowly but surely, how to help that process along. Despite our fears, the future beckons and holds much hope for all of us!

Resources

Websites, Magazines, and Newsletters

GENERAL INFORMATION ON ADHD

U.S. Centers for Disease Control and Prevention

The CDC has an authoritative site dedicated to ADHD.

www.cdc.gov/ncbddd/adhd

U.S. National Institute of Mental Health

The NIMH provides an authoritative summary of facts about ADHD.

www.nimh.nih.gov/health/topics/attention-deficit-hyperactivity-disorder-adhd/index.shtml

FURTHER INFORMATION ON ADHD, CHILDREN'S HEALTH AND DEVELOPMENT, AND PARENT AND FAMILY SUPPORT

CHADD (Child and Adults with Attention Deficit Disorder)

CHADD is a national family-support organization that hosts meetings and also has information on its web page; you may find local chapters in some communities. They also publish *ATTENTION!* magazine with practical articles, advice, and updates and organize an annual conference.

www.chadd.org/default.aspx

National Alliance on Mental Illness

NAMI historically was a support organization for individuals with severe mental illness and their families but now provides peer-to-peer support for a very wide range of conditions including ADHD, depression, and others, including groups for those affected and for family members. Many states have local chapters that may run support groups in your community; they are listed on the group's website.

www.nami.org

ADDitude

Another support option for families and sufferers is provided by the magazine and website called *ADDitude*. Every issue includes articles on a range of topics, many of which include comments from leading experts in the field. They also offer webinars and other resources.

www.additudemag.com

Russell A. Barkley, PhD, publishes a regular newsletter that you can subscribe to in print or online and includes summaries of recent science.

http://russellbarkley.org/newsletter.html

Psychiatric Times

Psychiatric Times is a monthly online publication offering feature articles, clinical news, and reports on special topics from expert writers across a broad range of psychiatric issues involving children and adults. Caution: You have to overlook extensive full-page ads for psychiatric medications while reading.

www.psychiatrictimes.com

American Academy of Pediatrics

The AAP is an excellent source of information about all aspects of children's health, including ADHD, and suggestions for children's use of technology.

www.aap.org

Canadian Paediatric Society

The CPS serves both CPS members and other health care professionals with information they need to make informed decisions about child health care. Parents, journalists, and others involved in the care of children will also find their website useful.

www.cps.ca

CanChild Centre for Childhood Disability Research

This research and educational center focuses on children and teenagers with physical, developmental, and communication needs and their families.

www.canchild.ca

Raising Children Network

This is a comprehensive website for Australian parents, offering resources, discussion forums, videos, and more, including information on teen development, learning difficulties, autism, and ADHD. Articles have age keys so parents and kids can read them.

http://raisingchildren.net.au

Centre for ADHD Awareness, Canada

CADDAC is the national support group for ADHD in Canada.

www.caddac.ca

BRAIN SCIENCE, GENETICS, AND EPIGENETICS

The Society for Neuroscience website provides a rich, accessible set of information modules for the general public at *www.brainfacts.org*.

The subscription magazine *Scientific American* covers new developments in cognitive neuroscience accessible to the layperson at *www.scientificamerican.com/mind*.

Brain Connection (*www.brainconnection.com*), sponsored by BrainHQ, a group promoting cognitive brain training, provides a variety of articles and resources about brain development and new brain research, including several articles on children's learning.

For information about CRISPR-CAS9 gene-editing technology, see this article on the *National Geographic* website: *www.nationalgeographic.com/magazine/2016/08/dna-crispr-gene-editing-science-ethics*.

The *Guardian* has put together a well-written lay summary of the key points of epigenetics at *www.theguardian.com/science/occams-corner/2014/apr/25/epigenetics-beginners-guide-to-everything*.

The National Institutes of Health (NIH) has a website for its epigenetics consortium that occasionally posts cutting-edge plans and breakthroughs (*http://ihec-epigenomes.org*) and also includes videos and tutorials (*http://ihec-epigenomes.org/why-epigenomics/video-clips*), as well as links to other resources under its "About" and "Why epigenomics" links.

An online course on epigenetics is offered by the University of Melbourne at *www.coursera.org/learn/epigenetics*.

NUTRITIONAL PLANNING FOR CHILDREN

For formal food allergies (not usually the case in ADHD but can occur), detailed suggestions and information for parents and educators are available at the CDC-sponsored site *www.foodallergy.org.*

Guidelines and tips for healthy nutritional planning for your child are available at the National Institutes of Health (*https://medlineplus.gov/childnutrition.html*) and the USDA (*http://fnic.nal.usda.gov/lifecycle-nutrition/child-nutrition*).

Several books written for the general public by members of the nutrition faculty at Harvard Medical School are listed at *http://nutrition.med.harvard.edu/publications.html.*

SLEEP PROBLEMS

The National Sleep Foundation provides background information, checklists, and guidelines at *https://sleepfoundation.org.*

Sleep behavioral programs are outlined at *http://drcraigcanapari.com/at-long-last-sleep-training-tools-for-the-exhausted-parent.*

EXERCISE PROGRAMS FOR KIDS

The U.S. Centers for Disease Control and Prevention provides clear guidelines, lists of activities that are moderate versus vigorous for different ages, and suggestions on getting activity into your child's life at *www.cdc.gov/physicalactivity/basics/children/index.htm.*

The CDC's Body and Mind (BAM!) website has interactive tools for you and your children and information on how to participate in dozens of different individual and group activities, games, and sports to help you identify suitable activities (*www.cdc.gov/bam/activity/index.html*).

If you are an educator looking for a health curriculum for children and families, check out the University of Texas CATCH (Coordinated Approach to Child Health) health curriculum, designed for schools and educators, which includes a family/home module (*http://catchinfo.org/about*).

TECHNOLOGY

Children's Technology Review provides professional reviews of interactive technology (software, videogames) at *www.childrenstech.com* to help guide parents and professionals in monitoring and choosing products that children are exposed to daily.

CHEMICAL TOXICANTS

The U.S. Environmental Protection Agency provides a thorough summary of how to protect your home from lead at *www.epa.gov/lead/protect-your-family-exposures-lead*.

Water filters should be certified for lead by NSF (*http://info.nsf.org/Certified/DWTU*), the Water Quality Association (*www.wqa.org*), or Underwriters Laboratories (*www.ul.com*).

The Northwest Center for Alternatives to Pesticides provides pest-specific ideas for safe pest control at *www.pesticide.org/resources_for_pests*.

The consumer-oriented Safer Chemicals, Healthy Families coalition provides information and suggestions on finding safe products on its website, *http://saferchemicals.org/category/find_safer_products*. In particular, note that the MADE SAFE label and the EPA label are recommended.

The *Huffington Post* offers several practical suggestions and lists companies that produce nontoxic children's products at *www.huffingtonpost.com/jamie-davis-smith/the-nontoxic-baby_b_5705873.html*.

STRESS AND TRAUMA

The National Child Traumatic Stress Network (NCTSN) website has a wealth of information to help you address your child's experience with traumatic stress at *www.nctsn.org*.

The CDC has a good summary of basic strategies to help you and your kids prevent or handle too much stress, as well as hotline and help numbers at *www.cdc.gov/violenceprevention/pub/coping_with_stress_tips.html*.

School-related resources and approaches for educators and professionals are listed at the Ohio University Center for Intervention Research in Schools: *www.oucirs.org/resources/educators-mh-professionals*.

PARENTING AND PARENT SUPPORT

Parents Magazine offers general advice on child development and parenting issues at *www.parents.com*.

Dr. Ross Greene's website provides collaborative solutions for parents and families, including helpful video clips, self-assessment checklists, and other resources at *www.livesinthebalance.org.*

The Massachusetts General Hospital website has a description of its similar program but less detail on resources: *www.thinkkids.org.*

The Yale Parenting Center offers parent management training using Alan Kazdin's modifications at *http://yaleparentingcenter.yale.edu.*

Carolyn Webster-Stratton's Incredible Years program, for young children (under age six), is supported by empirical studies; while primarily geared toward classroom use by educators, the website includes handouts and books for parents at *http://incredibleyears.com/parents-teachers/for-parents.*

Also for young children, Zero to Three (*www.zerotothree.org*) provides information on a host of topics (brain development, nutrition, child rearing) for adults who influence the lives of infants and toddlers.

MyADHD (*www.myadhd.com*) is a subscription website that offers tools for assessment, treatment, and progress monitoring, as well as a library of articles, audio programs, and charts that parents can use to better understand and manage their child's attention disorder.

The National Institute of Child Health and Human Development has a wealth of general information on child development for parents at *www.nichd.nih.gov/audiences/parents/Pages/home.aspx.*

TREATMENT GUIDELINES

Official treatment guidelines for ADHD are slightly different in Europe, Great Britain, and the United States.

Europe

European guidelines: *www.adhd-institute.com/disease-management/guidelines/european-guidelines*

United Kingdom: NICE guidelines are available at *www.nice.org.uk/Guidance/QS39.* For an expert overview of the guidelines go to *http://addiss.co.uk/NICE%20Guidelines.pdf.*

United States

American Academy of Pediatrics (accessible discussion and summary of AAP guidelines on the CDC website): *www.cdc.gov/ncbddd/adhd/guidelines.html*

American Academy of Child and Adolescent Psychiatry (AACAP) practice parameters for ADHD: *www.jaacap.com/article/S0890-8567(09)62182-1/ pdf*. Other AACAP guidelines for selected conditions: *www.aacap.org/aacap/ resources_for_primary_care/practice_parameters_and_resource_centers/practice_ parameters.aspx.*

EVIDENCE–BASED AND ALTERNATIVE TREATMENTS

A list of organizations that provide information on evidence-based practices is at *www.samhsa.gov/ebp-web-guide/mental-health-treatment.*

The Society of Clinical Child and Adolescent Psychology has a website that offers information on evidence-based mental health treatment for children and adolescents at *http://effectivechildtherapy.org.*

Books for Further Reading

ADHD

Banaschewski, T., Zuddas, A., Asherson, P., Buitelaar, J., Coghill, D., Danckaerts, M., et al. (2015). *ADHD and hyperkinetic disorder* (2nd ed.). Oxford, UK: Oxford University Press. While written as a practical guide for mental health professionals, this series of chapters by different experts in the field can also provide an advanced tutorial for sufficiently prepared members of the general public.

Barkley, R. A. (2014). *Attention-deficit hyperactivity disorder: A handbook for diagnosis and treatment* (4th ed.). New York: Guilford Press. A comprehensive explanation of what is known about ADHD, its history, and treatment approaches explained by leading experts in the field. With a focus on history, assessment, and standard treatments (school, parent counseling, medications), it also includes excellent chapters on nutrition and alternative treatments.

Brown, T. E. (2013). *A new understanding of ADHD in children and adults: Executive function impairments.* New York: Routledge. This readable yet scholarly book provides a description of ADHD using the lens of executive functioning.

Hinshaw, S., & Ellison, K. (2016). *ADHD: What everyone needs to know.* Oxford, UK: Oxford University Press. Brief, one- to two-page answers to dozens of common questions about ADHD in easy-to-read terms.

Nadeau, K. G., Littman, E. B., & Quinn, P. O. (2015). *Understanding girls with ADHD*. Silver Spring, MD: Advantage Books. A well-conceived summary of the particular issues that may face girls with ADHD, an understudied topic by educators who have spent their career studying attention and learning issues.

Nigg, J. T. (2006). *What causes ADHD?: Understanding what goes wrong and why*. New York: Guilford Press. A summary of multiple aspects of ADHD causality, including basic brain networks, genetic influences, and more detail on the research linking ADHD to different gene × environment interactions.

PARENTING AND PARENT SUPPORT

Barkley, R. A. (2013). *Taking charge of ADHD: The complete authoritative guide for parents* (3rd ed.). New York: Guilford Press. A practical guide from a renowned authority that includes a behavior management plan.

Barkley, R. A., & Benton, C. M. (2013). *Your defiant child: Eight steps to better behavior* (2nd ed.). New York: Guilford Press. Practical explanation of how to apply well-understood behavioral principles to build your child's sense of responsibility.

Forehand, R., & Long, N. (2010). *Parenting the strong-willed child*. New York: McGraw-Hill Education. An expert summary of the steps and skills to managing an obstinate youngster from leaders in the field.

Greene, R. (2014). *The explosive child: A new approach for understanding and parenting easily frustrated, chronically inflexible children*. New York: Harper. Revised and updated edition of a classic. Greene, a leader in developing collaborative, innovative approaches to working with children and parenting, tackles some of the most difficult child behaviors—tantrums, meltdowns, hitting, spitting—with well-thought-out practical suggestions related to his collaborative approach.

Kazdin, A. (2009). *The Kazdin method for parenting the defiant child*. Boston: Mariner Books.

Kazdin, A., & Rotella, C. (2014). *The everyday parenting toolkit*. Boston: Mariner Books. Both of Alan Kazdin's authoritative, yet very practical, easy-to-use books for parents are full of practical skills, stories, and specific guidelines for how to solve common parenting problems. Kazdin encourages an engaged, positive, reward-based approach to helping children get on track and tackles everyday problems from sleep routine to interrupting to misbehavior in public with practical steps.

Webster-Stratton, C. (2005). *The incredible years: A troubleshooting guide for parents of children aged 2–8*. Seattle: Incredible Years. A practical guide from one of the top experts and innovators on application of behavioral management approaches to young children. It can be ordered through her website *http://incredibleyears.com/books/the-incredible-years-guide*

BRAIN DEVELOPMENT

Galinsky, E. (2010). *Mind in the making: The seven essential life skills every child needs.* New York: HarperStudio. A readable summary of priorities for developing children's practical life skills, coping, and regulation based on neuroscience.

Kahneman, D. (2011). *Thinking fast and slow.* New York: Farrar, Straus and Giroux. A delightful and accessible explanation from Nobel Prize winner and expert cognitive psychologist Daniel Kahneman, often credited with launching the field of behavioral economics. Includes explanations of automatic and controlled processing, and the automatic decision-making intuitions (heuristics) that sometimes lead us to make "illogical" choices.

EPIGENETICS

Moore, D. S. (2015). *The developing genome: An introduction to behavioral epigenetics.* New York: Oxford University Press. This book, which has won the American Psychological Association's annual book award, provides an excellent and intelligent explanation for the general public.

NUTRITION

Lenkert, E., & Alpert, B. London: Kyle Books. *Healthy eating during pregnancy.* Includes extended discussion of breastfeeding, as well as feeding guidelines for infants and toddlers and school-age children, as well as discussion of school lunches, sports drinks, and more.

Walker, W. A. (2006). *Eat, play, and be healthy: The Harvard Medical School guide to healthy eating for kids.* New York: McGraw-Hill. This book aims to answer children's nutrition questions and includes tips and specific food plans and recipes. Also comes as an abridged CD on Amazon.

EXERCISE

Ratey, J. J., & Hagerman, E. (2013). *Spark: The revolutionary science of exercise and the brain.* New York: Little, Brown. Ratey's book will inspire and motivate you like no other to get engaged and put exercise back in your life and your child's life.

STRESS AND TRAUMA

Hayes, S. C., & Smith, S. (2005). *Get out of your mind and into your life.* Oakland, CA: New Harbinger. A self-help workbook to help you enhance coping skills.

Van der Kolk, B. (2014). *The body keeps score: Brain, mind and body in the healing of trauma.* New York: Viking. A comprehensive yet accessible summary of the psychological, biological, and physical consequences of psychological trauma and the associated toxic stress response, complete with the latest thinking on treatment, from one of the world's leading researchers on trauma effects.

Williams, M., Teasdale, J., Segal, Z., & Kabat-Zinn, J. (2007). *The mindful way through depression.* New York: Guilford Press. The classic application of mindfulness in a self-help format for mood and depression.

ORGANIZATIONAL AND EXECUTIVE SKILLS TRAINING FOR KIDS

Dawson, P., & Guare, R. (2009). *Smart but scattered.* New York: Guilford Press. A resource and workbook for parents to help children develop executive function skills, filled with practical tips and handy worksheets.

Gallagher, R., & Abikoff, H. (2014). *Organizational skills training for children with ADHD: An empirically supported treatment.* New York: Guilford Press. A formal curriculum for organizational skills training explained; this could be followed at home by parents, probably with some advice from a counselor or knowledgeable special education teacher.

References

The following are the key sources for the studies mentioned and research findings discussed in the text.

CHAPTER 1: A NEW UNDERSTANDING OF ADHD

Banich, M. T. (2009). Executive function: The search for an integrated account. *Current Directions in Psychological Science, 18*(2), 89–94.

Barkley, R. A. (2012). *Executive functions: What they are, how they work, and why they evolved.* New York: Guilford Press.

Baumeister, R. F., Vohs, K. D., & Tice, D. M. (2007). The strength model of self-control. *Current Directions in Psychological Science, 16*(6), 351–355.

Becker S. P., Leopold, D. R., Burns, G. L., Jarrett, M. A., Langberg, J. M., Marshall, S. A., et al. (2016). The internal, external, and diagnostic validity of sluggish cognitive tempo: A meta-analysis and critical review. *Journal of the American Academy of Child and Adolescent Psychiatry, 55*(3), 163–178.

Bertrams, A., Baumeister, R. F., & Englert, C. (2016). Higher self-control capacity predicts lower anxiety-impaired cognition during math examinations. *Frontiers of Psychology, 31*(7), 485.

Botvinick, M., & Braver, T. (2015). Motivation and cognitive control: From behavior to neural mechanism. *Annual Review of Psychology, 66*, 83–113.

Carter, E. C., Pedersen, E. J., & McCullough, M. E. (2015). Reassessing intertemporal choice: Human decision-making is more optimal in a foraging task than in a self-control task. *Frontiers in Psychology, 6*, 95.

de Ridder, D. T., Lensvelt-Mulders, G., Finkenauer, C., Stok, F. M., & Baumeister, R. F. (2012). Taking stock of self-control: A meta-analysis of how trait self-control relates to a wide range of behaviors. *Personality and Social Psychology Review, 16*(1), 76–99.

Diamond, A. (2013). Executive functions. *Annual Review of Psychology, 64*, 135–168.

Evans, J. S. (2008). Dual-processing accounts of reasoning, judgment, and social cognition. *Annual Review of Psychology, 59*, 255–278.

Graziano, P. A., & Garcia, A. (2016). Attention-deficit hyperactivity disorder and children's emotion dysregulation: A meta-analysis. *Clinical Psychology Review*, 46, 106–123.

Groen-Blokhuis, M. M., Middeldorp, C. M., Kan, K. J., Abdellaoui, A., van Beijsterveldt, C. E., Ehli, E. A., et al. (2014). Attention-deficit/hyperactivity disorder polygenic risk scores predict attention problems in a population-based sample of children. *Journal of the American Academy of Child and Adolescent Psychiatry*, 53(10), 1123–1129.

Huang-Pollock, C., Ratcliff, R., McKoon, G., Shapiro, Z., Weigard, A., & Galloway-Long, H. (2017). Using the diffusion model to explain cognitive deficits in attention deficit hyperactivity disorder. *Journal of Abnormal Child Psychology*, 45, 57–68.

Karalunas, S. L., Geurts, H. M., Konrad, K., Bender, S., & Nigg, J. T. (2014). Annual research review: Reaction time variability in ADHD and autism spectrum disorders: Measurement and mechanisms of a proposed trans-diagnostic phenotype. *Journal of Child Psychology and Psychiatry*, 55(6), 685–710.

Lahey, B. B., Applegate, B., Hakes, J. K., Zald, D. H., Hariri, A. R., & Rathouz, P. J. (2012). Is there a general factor of prevalent psychopathology during adulthood? *Journal of Abnormal Psychology*, 121(4), 971–977.

McLoughlin, G., Albrecht, B., Banaschewski, T., Rothenburger, A., Brandeis, D., Asherson, P., et al (2010). Electrophysiological evidence for abnormal preparatory states and inhibitory processing in adult ADHD. *Behavioral and Brain Functions*, 6(66).

Mead, N. L., Baumeister, R. F., Gino, F., Schweitzer, M. E., & Ariely, D. (2009). Too tired to tell the truth: Self-control resource depletion and dishonesty. *Journal of Experimental Social Psychology*, 45(3), 594–597.

Miller, E. K., & Buschman, T. J. (2012). Top-down control of attention by rhythmic neural computations. In M. I. Posner (Ed.), *Cognitive neuroscience of attention* (2nd ed., pp. 229–241). New York: Guilford Press.

Nigg, J. T. (2013). Attention-deficit/hyperactivity disorder and adverse health outcomes. *Clinical Psychology Review*, 33, 215–228.

Nigg, J. T. (2016). Inattention and impulsivity. In D. Cicchetti (Ed.), *Developmental psychopathology* (3rd ed.): Vol. 3. *Maladaptation and psychopathology* (pp. 591–646). New York: Wiley.

Nigg, J. T. (2017). Annual research review: On the relations between self-regulation, executive function, cognitive control, effortful control, impulsivity, risk taking, and response inhibition in developmental psychopathology. *Journal of Child Psychology and Psychiatry*, 58(4), 361–383.

Petersen, S. E., & Posner, M. I. (2012). The attention system of the human brain: 20 years after. *Annual Review of Neuroscience*, 35, 73–89.

Rothbart, M. K. (2011). *Becoming who we are: Temperament and personality in development*. New York: Guilford Press.

Shaw, P., Stringaris, A., Nigg, J., & Leibenluft, E. (2014). Emotion dysregulation in attention deficit hyperactivity disorder. *American Journal of Psychiatry*, 171(3), 276–293.

Sonuga-Barke, E., Bitsakou, P., & Thompson, M. (2010). Beyond the dual pathway model: Evidence for the dissociation of timing, inhibitory, and delay-related impairments in attention-deficit/hyperactivity disorder. *Journal of the American Academy of Child and Adolescent Psychiatry, 49*(4), 345–355.

Tangney, J. P., Baumeister, R. F., & Boone, A. L. (2004). High self-control predicts good adjustment, less pathology, better grades, and interpersonal success. *Journal of Personality, 72*(2), 271–324.

Verbruggen, F., McLaren, I. P. L., & Chambers, C. D. (2014). Banishing the control homunculi in studies of action control and behavior change. *Perspectives on Psychological Science, 9*, 497–524.

Zelazo, P. D., & Carlson, S. M. (2012). Hot and cool executive function in childhood and adolescence: Development and plasticity. *Child Development Perspectives, 6*(4), 354–360.

CHAPTER 2: EPIGENETICS: THE END OF THE NATURE–VERSUS–NURTURE DEBATE

Adisetiyo, V., Tabesh, A., Di Martino, A., Falangola, M. F., Castellanos, F. X., Jensenk J. H., et al. (2014). Attention-deficit/hyperactivity disorder without comorbidity is associated with distinct atypical patterns of cerebral microstructural development. *Human Brain Mapping, 35*(5), 2148–2162.

Babenko, O., Kovalchuk, I., & Metz, G. A. (2015). Stress-induced perinatal and transgenerational epigenetic programming of brain development and mental health. *Neuroscience and Biobehavioral Reviews, 48*, 70–91.

Bale, T. L. (2015). Epigenetic and transgenerational reprogramming of brain development. *Nature Reviews: Neuroscience, 16*(6), 332–344.

Belsky, J., Pluess, M., & Widaman, K. F. (2013). Confirmatory and competitive evaluation of alternative gene–environment interaction hypotheses. *Journal of Child Psychology and Psychiatry and Allied Disciplines, 54*(10), 1135–1143.

Berger, S. L., Kouzarides, T., Shiekhattar, R., & Shilatifard, A. (2009). An operational definition of epigenetics. *Genes and Development, 23*(7), 781–783.

Bolton, J. L., & Bilbo, S. D. (2014). Developmental programming of brain and behavior by perinatal diet: Focus on inflammatory mechanisms. *Dialogues in Clinical Neuroscience, 16*(3), 307–320.

Burt, S. A. (2009). Rethinking environmental contributions to child and adolescent psychopathology: A meta-analysis of shared environmental influences. *Psychological Bulletin, 135*(4), 608–637.

Byrd, A. L., & Manuck, S. B. (2014). MAO-A, childhood maltreatment, and antisocial behavior: Meta-analysis of a gene-environment interaction. *Biological Psychiatry, 75*(1), 9–17.

Castellanos, F. X., & Proal, E. (2012). Large-scale brain systems in ADHD: Beyond the prefrontal–striatal model. *Trends in Cognitive Sciences, 16*(1), 17–26.

Castellanos, F. X., Sharp, W. S., Gottesman, R. F., Greenstein, D. K., Giedd, J. N., & Rapoport, J. L. (2003). Anatomic brain abnormalities in monozygotic twins discordant for attention deficit hyperactivity disorder. *American Journal of Psychiatry, 160*(9), 1693–1696.

Di Martino, A., Fair, D. A., Kelly, C., Satterthwaite, T. D., Castellanos, F. X., Thomason, M. E., et al. (2014). Unraveling the miswired connectome: A developmental perspective. *Neuron, 83*(6), 1335–1353.

Dolinov, D. C., Huang, D., & Jirtle, R. L. (2007). Maternal nutrient supplementation counteracts bisphenol A-induced DNA hypomethylation in early development. *Proceedings of the National Academy of Science, 104*(32), 13056–13061.

Ellis, B. J., Boyce, W. T., Belsky, J., Bakermans-Kranenburg, M. J., & van IJzendoorn, M. H. (2011). Differential susceptibility to the environment: An evolutionary-neurodevelopmental theory. *Development and Psychopathology, 23*(1), 7–28.

Elmore, A. L., Nigg, J. T., Friderici, K. H., & Nikolas, M. A. (2016). Does 5HTTLPR genotype moderate the association of family environment with child attention-deficit hyperactivity disorder symptomatology? *Journal of Clinical Child and Adolescent Psychology, 45*(3), 348–360.

Fair, D. A., Bathula, D., Nikolas, M. A., & Nigg, J. T. (2012). Distinct neuropsychological subgroups in typically developing youth inform heterogeneity in children with ADHD. *Proceedings of the National Academy of Sciences of the United States of America, 109*(17), 6769–6774.

Goodkind, M., Eickhoff, S. B., Oathes, D. J., Jiang, Y., Chang, A., Jones-Hagata, L., et al. (2015). Identification of a common neurobiological substrate for mental illness. *Journal American Medical Association Psychiatry, 72*(4), 305–315.

Insel, T., Cuthbert, B., Garvey, M., Heinssen, R., Pine, D. S., Quinn, K., et al. (2010). Research domain criteria (rdoc): Toward a new classification framework for research on mental disorders. *American Journal of Psychiatry, 167*(7), 748–751.

Iyegbe, C., Campbell, D., Butler, A., Ajnakina, O., & Sham, P. (2014). The emerging molecular architecture of schizophrenia, polygenic risk scores and the clinical implications for gxe research. *Social Psychiatry and Psychiatric Epidemiology, 49*(2), 169–182.

Karalunas, S. L., Fair, D., Musser, E. D., Aykes, K., Iyer, S. P., & Nigg, J. T. (2014). Subtyping attention-deficit/hyperactivity disorder using temperament dimensions: Toward biologically based nosologic criteria. *Journal of the American Medical Association: Psychiatry, 71*(9), 1015–1024.

Lahey, B. B., Van Hulle, C. A., Singh, A. L., Waldman, I. D., & Rathouz, P. J. (2011). Higher-order genetic and environmental structure of prevalent forms of child and adolescent psychopathology. *Archives of General Psychiatry, 68*(2), 181–189.

Lee, S. H., Ripke, S., Neale, B. M., Faraone, S. V., Purcell, S. M., Perlis, R. H., et al. (2013). Genetic relationship between five psychiatric disorders estimated from genome-wide snps. *Nature Genetics, 45*(9), 984–994.

Lu, Y. F., & Menard, S. (2016). The interplay of MAOA and peer influences in predicting adult criminal behavior. *Psychiatry Quarterly, 88*(1), 115–128.

Ma, B., Wilker, E. H., Willis-Owen, S. A., Byun, H. M., Wong, K. C., Motta, V., et al. (2014). Predicting DNA methylation level across human tissues. *Nucleic Acids Research, 42*(6), 3515–3528.

Martin, J., O'Donovan, M. C., Thapar, A., Langley, K., & Williams, N. (2015). The relative contribution of common and rare genetic variants to ADHD. *Translational Psychiatry, 5*(2), e506.

McPherson, N. O., Bell, V. G., Zander-Fox, D. L., Fullston, T., Wu, L. L., Robker,

R. L., et al. (2015). When two obese parents are worse than one!: Impacts on embryo and fetal development. *American Journal of Physiology: Endocrinology and Metabolism, 309*(6), E568–E581.

Middeldorp, C. M., Hammerschlag, A. R., Ouwens, K. G., Groen-Blokhuis, M. M., St Pourcain, B., Greven, C. U., et al. (2016). A genome-wide association meta-analysis of attention-deficit/hyperactivity disorder symptoms in population-based pediatric cohorts. *Journal of the American Academy of Child and Adolescent Psychiatry, 55*(10), 896–905.

Miller, A. H., & Raison, C. L. (2015). Are anti-inflammatory therapies viable treatments for psychiatric disorders?: Where the rubber meets the road. *Journal of the American Medical Association: Psychiatry, 72*(6), 527–528.

Morgan et al. (2016). Parental serotonin transporter polymorphism (5-HTTLPR) moderates associations of stress and child behavior with parenting behavior. *Journal of Clinical Child and Adolescent Psychology, 18*, 1–12.

Nigg, J. T. (2016). Where do epigenetics and developmental origins take the field of developmental psychopathology? *Journal of Abnormal Child Psychology, 44*(3), 405–419.

Nigg, J. T. Nikolas, M., & Burt, S. A. (2010). Measured gene by environment interaction in relation to attention-deficit/hyperactivity disorder (ADHD). *Journal of the American Academy of Child and Adolescent Psychiatry, 49*, 863–873.

Petrill, S. A., Bartlett, C. W., & Blair, C. (2013). Gene–environment interplay in child psychology and psychiatry—challenges and ways forward. *Journal of Child Psychology and Psychiatry and Allied Disciplines, 54*(10), 1029.

Psychiatric Genetics Consortium Cross Disorder Group. (2013). Identification of risk loci with shared effects on five major psychiatric disorders: A genome-wide analysis. *Lancet, 81*(9875), 1371–1379.

Purcell, S. (2002). Variance components models for gene–environment interaction in twin analysis. *Twin Research, 5*(6), 554–571.

Ray, S., Miller, M., Karalunas, S., Robertson, C., Grayson, D. S., Cary, R. P., et al. (2014). Structural and functional connectivity of the human brain in autism spectrum disorders and attention-deficit/hyperactivity disorder: A rich club-organization study. *Human Brain Mapping, 35*(12), 6032–6048.

Sharma, S., Powers, A., Bradley, B., & Ressler, K. J. (2016). Gene × environment determinants of stress- and anxiety-related disorders. *Annual Review of Psychology, 67*, 239–216.

Sharpley, C. F., Palanisamy, S. K., Glyde, N. S., Dillingham, P. W., & Agnew, L. L. (2014, October). An update on the interaction between the serotonin transporter promoter variant (5-HTTLPR), stress and depression, plus an exploration of non-confirming findings. *Behavioral Brain Research, 273*(15), 89–105.

Shaw, P., Lerch, J., Greenstein, D., Sharp, W., Clasen, L., Evans, A., et al. (2006). Longitudinal mapping of cortical thickness and clinical outcome in children and adolescents with attention-deficit/hyperactivity disorder. *Archives of General Psychiatry, 63*(5), 540–549.

Sng, J., & Meaney, M. J. (2009). Environmental regulation of the neural epigenome. *Epigenomics, 1*(1), 131–151.

Stergiakouli, E., Martin, J., Hamshere, M. L., Langley, K., Evans, D. M., St Pour-
    cain, B., et al. (2015). Shared genetic influences between attention-deficit/
    hyperactivity disorder (ADHD) traits in children and clinical ADHD. *Journal
    of the American Academy of Child and Adolescent Psychiatry, 54*(4), 322–327.
Szyf, M., & Bick, J. (2013). DNA methylation: A mechanism for embedding early
    life experiences in the genome. *Child Development, 84,* 49–57.
van IJzendoorn, M. H., Belsky, J., & Bakermans-Kranenburg, M. J. (2012). Sero-
    tonin transporter genotype 5HTTLPR as a marker of differential suscepti-
    bility?: A meta-analysis of child and adolescent gene-by-environment studies.
    Translational Psychiatry, 2, e147.
Wang, Q., Yang, C., Gelernter, J., & Zhao, H. (2015). Pervasive pleiotropy between
    psychiatric disorders and immune disorders revealed by integrative analysis of
    multiple GWAS. *Human Genetics, 134*(11–12), 1195–1209.
Wilmot, B., Fry, R., Smeester, L., Musser, E. D., Mill, J., & Nigg, J. T. (2016). Methy-
    lomic analysis of salivary DNA in childhood ADHD. *Journal of Child Psychol-
    ogy and Psychiatry, 57,* 152–160.
Zhu, T., Gan, J., Huang, J., Li, Y., Qu, Y., & Mu, D. J. (2016). Association between
    perinatal hypoxic-ischemic conditions and attention-deficit/hyperactivity dis-
    order: A meta-analysis. *Journal of Child Neurology, 31,* 1235–1244.

CHAPTER 3: FOOD AND ADHD: OLD CONTROVERSIES AND NEW CLARITY

Access to sanitation. United Nations Department of Economic and Social Affairs.
    Retrieved June 15, 2006, from *www.un.org/waterforlifedecade/sanitation.shtml.*
Arnold, L. E., Hurt, E., & Lofthouse, N. (2013). Attention-deficit/hyperactivity
    disorder: Dietary and nutritional treatments. *Child and Adolescent Psychiatric
    Clinics of North America, 22*(3), 381–402.
Bubnov, R. V., Spivak, M. Y., Lazarenko, L. M., Bomba, A., & Boyko, N. V. (2015).
    Probiotics and immunity: Provisional role for personalized diets and disease
    prevention. *EPMA Journal, 6*(1), 14.
Caso, J. R., Balanzá-Martínez, V., Palomo, T., & García-Bueno, B. (2016). The
    microbiota and gut-brain axis: Contributions to the immunopathogenesis of
    schizophrenia. *Current Pharmaceutical Design, 22,* 6122–6133.
Faraone, S. V., & Antshel, K. M. (2014). Towards an evidence-based taxonomy
    of nonpharmacologic treatments for ADHD. *Child and Adolescent Psychiatric
    Clinics of North America, 23*(4), 965–972.
Foster, J. A., Lyte, M., Meyer, E., & Cryan, J. F. (2016, April 29). Gut microbiota
    and brain function: An evolving field in neuroscience. *International Journal of
    Neuropsychopharmacology, 19*(5), pyv114.
Grayson, D. S., Kroenke, C. D., Neuringer, M., & Fair, D. A. (2014). Dietary
    omega-3 fatty acids modulate large-scale systems organization in the rhesus
    macaque brain. *Journal of Neuroscience, 34*(6), 2065–2074.
Hariri, M., & Azadbakht, L. (2015). Magnesium, iron, and zinc supplementation for
    the treatment of attention deficit hyperactivity disorder: A systematic review
    on the recent literature. *International Journal of Preventive Medicine, 6,* 83.

Hawkey, E., & Nigg, J. T. (2014). Omega-3 fatty acid and ADHD: Blood level analysis and meta-analytic extension of supplementation trials. *Clinical Psychology Review, 34*(6), 496–505.

Hurt, E. A., & Arnold, L. E. (2014). An integrated dietary/nutritional approach to ADHD. *Child and Adolescent Psychiatric Clinics of North America, 23*(4), 955–964.

Ioannidis, K., Chamberlain, S. R., & Müller, U. (2014). Ostracising caffeine from the pharmacological arsenal for attention-deficit hyperactivity disorder—was this a correct decision?: A literature review. *Journal of Psychopharmacology, 28*(9), 830–836.

Lusardi, T. A., Akula, K. K., Coffman, S. Q., Ruskin, D. N., Masino, S. A, & Boison D. (2015). Ketogenic diet prevents epileptogenesis and disease progression in adult mice and rats. *Neuropharmacology, 99*, 500–509.

Maqsood, R., & Stone, T. W. (2016). The gut-brain axis, BDNF, NMDA and CNS disorders. *Neurochemical Resesarch, 11*, 2819–2835.

Mayer, E. A., Tillisch, K., & Gupta, A. (2015). Gut/brain axis and the microbiota. *Journal of Clinical Investigation, 125*(3), 926–938.

Mittal, R., Debs, L. H., Patel, A. P., Nguyen, D., Patel, K., O'Connor, G., et al. (2016). Neurotransmitters: The critical modulators regulating gut-brain axis. *Journal of Cell Physiology.* [Epub ahead of print]

Mychasiuk, R., Hehar, H., Ma, I., & Esser, M. J. (2015, February 5). Dietary intake alters behavioral recovery and gene expression profiles in the brain of juvenile rats that have experienced a concussion. *Frontiers in Behavioral Neuroscience, 9*(17).

Nigg, J. T., & Holton, K. (2014). Restriction and Elimination diets in ADHD treatment. *Journal of Child and Adolescent Psychiatric Clinics of North America, 738*, 937–953.

Nigg, J. T., Lewis, K., Edinger, T., & Falk, M. (2012). Meta-analysis of ADHD or ADHD symptoms, restriction diet, and synthetic food color additives. *Journal of the American Academy of Child and Adolescent Psychiatry, 51*, 86–97.

Petra, A. I., Panagiotidou, S., Hatziagelaki, E., Stewart, J. M., Conti, P., & Theoharides, T. C. (2015). Gut-microbiota-brain axis and its effect on neuropsychiatric disorders with suspected immune dysregulation. *Clinical Therapeutics, 37*(5), 984–995.

Sable, P., Randhir, K., Kale, A., Chavan-Gautam, P., & Joshi, S. (2015). Maternal micronutrients and brain global methylation patterns in the offspring. *Nutritional Neuroscience, 18*(1), 30–36.

Stevens, L. J., Kuczek T., Burgess, J. R., Hurt, E., & Arnold, L. E. (2011). Dietary sensitivities and ADHD symptoms: Thirty-five years of research. *Clinical Pediatrics, 50*(4), 279–293.

Stevenson, J., Buitelaar, J., Cortese, S., Ferrin, M., Konofal, E., Lecendreux, M., et al. (2014). Research review: The role of diet in the treatment of attention-deficit/hyperactivity disorder—an appraisal of the evidence on efficacy and recommendations on the design of future studies. *Journal of Child Psychology and Psychiatry, 55*(5), 416–427.

Stevenson, J., Sonuga-Barke, E., McCann, D., Grimshaw, K., Parker, K. M., Rose-Zerilli, M. J., et al. (2010). The role of histamine degradation gene polymorphisms in moderating the effects of food additives on children's ADHD symptoms. *American Journal of Psychiatry, 167*(9), 1108–1115.

Sullivan, E. L., Nousen, E. K., & Chamlou, K. A. (2014). Maternal high fat diet consumption during the perinatal period programs offspring behavior. *Physiology and Behavior, 123,* 236–242.

Wolraich, M. L., Wilson, D. B., & White, J. W. (1995). The effect of sugar on behavior or cognition in children: A meta-analysis. *Journal of the American Medical Association, 274*(20), 1617–1621.

World Health Organization and UNICEF Joint Monitoring Programme (JMP). (2015). Progress on sanitation and drinking water: 2015 update and MDG assessment. Available at *www.who.int/water_sanitation_health/monitoring/jmp-2015-update/en.*

Yarandi, S. S., Peterson, D. A., Treisman, G. J., Moran, T. H., & Pasricha, P. J. (2016). Modulatory effects of gut microbiota on the central nervous system: How gut could play a role in neuropsychiatric health and diseases. *Journal of Neurogastroenterology and Motility, 22*(2), 201–212.

CHAPTER 4: EXERCISE, SLEEP, AND ADHD: NEW INSIGHTS ON BRAIN GROWTH

Archer, T., & Kostrzewa, R. M. (2015). Physical exercise alleviates health defects, symptoms, and biomarkers in schizophrenia spectrum disorder. *Neurotoxicity Research, 28*(3), 268–280.

Auger, R. R., Burgess, H. J., Emens, J. S., Deriy, L. V., Thomas, S. M., & Sharkey, K. M. (2015). Clinical practice guideline for the treatment of intrinsic circadian rhythm sleep-wake disorders: Advanced sleep-wake phase disorder (ASWPD), delayed sleep-wake phase disorder (DSWPD), non-24-hour sleep-wake rhythm disorder (N24SWD), and irregular ake rhythm disorder (ISWRD). *Journal of Clinical Sleep Medicine, 11*(10), 1199–1236.

Barnes, C. M., & Drake C. L. (2015). Prioritizing sleep health: Public health policy recommendations. *Perspectives on Psychological Science, 10*(6), 733–737.

Bruni, O., Alonso-Alconada, D., Besag, F., Biran, V., Braam, W., Cortese, S., et al. (2015). Current role of melatonin in pediatric neurology: Clinical recommendations. *European Journal of Paediatric Neurology, 19*(2), 122–133.

Burdette, H. L., & Whitaker, R. C. (2005). Resurrecting free play in young children: Looking beyond fitness and fatness to attention, affiliation, and affect. *Archives of Pediatric and Adolescent Medicine, 159*(1), 46–50.

Chang, A. M., Aeschbach, D., Duffy, J. F., & Czeisler, C. A. (2015). Evening use of light-emitting eReaders negatively affects sleep, circadian timing, and next-morning alertness. *Proceedings of the National Academy of Sciences, 112,* 1232–1237.

Den Heijer, A. E., Groen, Y., Tucha, L., Feuermaier, A. B. M., Koerts, J., Lange, K. W., et al. (2016, July 11). Sweat it out?: The effects of physical exercise on cognition and behavior in children and adults with ADHD: A systematic literature review. *Journal of Neural Transmission, 124*(Suppl. 1), 3–26.

Denham, J., Marques, F. Z., O'Brien, B. J., & Charchar, F. J. (2014). Exercise: Putting action into our epigenome. *Sports Medicine, 44*(2), 189–209.

Díaz-Román, A., Hita-Yáñez, E., & Buela-Casal, G. (2016). Sleep characteristics in children with attention deficit hyperactivity disorder: Systematic review and meta-analyses. *Journal of Clinical Sleep Medicine, 12*(5), 747–756.

Falbe, J., Davison, K. K., Franckle, R. L., Ganter, C., Gortmaker, S. L., Smith, L., et al. (2015). Sleep duration, restfulness, and screens in the sleep environment. *Pediatrics, 135*(2), e367–e375.

Gómez, R. L., & Edgin, J. O. (2015). Sleep as a window into early neural development: Shifts in sleep-dependent learning effects across early childhood. *Child Development Perspectives, 9*(3), 183–189.

Hackney, A. C. (2015). Epigenetic aspects of exercise on stress reactivity. *Psychoneuroendocrinology, 61,* 17.

Halperin, J. M., Berwid, O. G., & O'Neill, S. (2014). Healthy body, healthy mind? The effectiveness of physical activity to treat ADHD in children. *Child and Adolescent Psychiatric Clinics of North America, 23,* 899–936.

Hargreaves, M. (2015). Exercise and gene expression. *Progress in Molecular Biology and Translational Science, 135,* 457–469.

Hillman, C. H. (2014). The relation of childhood physical activity and aerobic fitness to brain function and cognition: A review. *Monographs of the Society for Research in Child Development, 79,* 1–6.

Horváth, K., Myers, K., Foster, R., & Plunkett, K. J. (2015). Napping facilitates word learning in early lexical development. *Sleep Research, 24*(5), 503–509.

Kashimoto, R. K., Toffoli, L. V., Manfredo, M. H., Volpini, V. L., Martins-Pinge, M. C., Pelosi, G. G., et al. (2016). Physical exercise affects the epigenetic programming of rat brain and modulates the adaptive response evoked by repeated restraint stress. *Behavioural Brain Research, 296,* 286–289.

Khan, N. A., & Hillman, C. H. (2014). Benefits of regular aerobic exercise for executive functioning in healthy populations. *Pediatric Exercise Science, 26,* 138–146.

Kidwell, K. M., Van Dyk, T. R., Lundahl, A., & Nelson, T. D. (2015). Stimulant medications and sleep for youth with ADHD: A meta-analysis. *Pediatrics, 136,* 1144–1153.

Maski, K. P. (2015). Sleep-dependent memory consolidation in children. *Seminars in Pediatric Neurology, 22*(2), 130–134.

Myer, G. D., Faigenbaum, A. D., Edwards, N. M., Clark, J. F., Best, T. M., & Sallis, R. E. (2015). Sixty minutes of what?: A developing brain perspective for activating children with an integrative exercise approach. *British Journal of Sports Medicine, 49*(23), 1510–1516.

Nelson, M. C., & Gordon-Larsen, P. (2006). Physical activity and sedentary behavior patterns are associated with selected adolescent health risk behaviors. *Pediatrics, 117,* 1281–1290.

Pan-Vazquez, A., Rye, N., Ameri, M., McSparron, B., Smallwood, G., Bickerdyke, J., et al. (2015). Impact of voluntary exercise and housing conditions on hippocampal glucocorticoid receptor, miR-124 and anxiety. *Molecular Brain, 8,* 40.

Rodrigues, G. M., Jr., Toffoli, L. V., Manfredo, M. H., Francis-Oliveira, J., Silva, A. S., Raquel, H. A., et al. (2015). Acute stress affects the global DNA methylation profile in rat brain: Modulation by physical exercise. *Behavioural Brain Research, 15*(279), 123–128.

Singh, A., Uijtdewilligen, L., Twisk, J. W., van Mechelen, W., & Chinapaw, M. J. (2012). Physical activity and performance at school: A systematic review of the literature including a methodological quality assessment. *Archives of Pediatric and Adolescent Medicine, 166*(1), 49–55.

Urbain, C., De Tiège, X., Op De Beeck, M., Bourguignon, M., Wens, V., Verheulpen D., et al. (2016). Sleep in children triggers rapid reorganization of memory-related brain processes. *NeuroImage, 134,* 213–222.

Vysniauske, R., Verburgh, L., Oosterlaan, J., & Molendijk, M. L. (2016). The effects of physical exercise on functional outcomes in the treatment of ADHD: A meta-analysis. *Journal of Attention Disorders.* [Epub ahead of print]

CHAPTER 5: TECHNOLOGY AND ADHD: LATEST FINDINGS ON THE PERIL AND THE PROMISE

Anderson, C. A., Berkowitz, L., Donnerstein, E., Huesmann, L. R., Johnson, J. D., Linz D., et al. (2003). The influence of media violence on youth. *Psychological Science in the Public Interest, 4*(3), 81–110.

Brevet-Aeby, C., Brunelin, J., Iceta, S., Padovan, C., & Poulet, E. (2016). Prefrontal cortex and impulsivity: Interest of noninvasive brain stimulation. *Neuroscience and Biobehavioral Reviews, 71,* 112–134.

Brunoni, A. R., & Vanderhasselt, M. A. (2014). Working memory improvement with non-invasive brain stimulation of the dorsolateral prefrontal cortex: A systematic review and meta-analysis. *Brain and Cognition, 86,* 1–9.

Bushman, B. J. (2016). Violent media and hostile appraisals: A meta-analytic review. *Aggressive Behavior, 42,* 605–613.

Bushman, B. J., & Anderson, C. A. (2001). Media violence and the American public: Scientific facts versus media misinformation. *American Psychologist, 56,* 477–489.

Cortese, S., Ferrin, M., Brandeis, D., Buitelaar, J., Daley, D., Dittmann, R. W., et al. (2015). Cognitive training for attention-deficit/hyperactivity disorder: Meta-analysis of clinical and neuropsychological outcomes from randomized controlled trials. *Journal of the American Academy of Child and Adolescent Psychiatry, 54*(3), 164–174.

Cortese, S., Ferrin, M., Brandeis, D., Holtmann, M., Aggensteiner, P., Daley, D., et al. (2016). Neurofeedback for attention-deficit/hyperactivity disorder: Meta-analysis of clinical and neuropsychological outcomes from randomized controlled trials. *Journal of the American Academy of Child and Adolescent Psychiatry, 55*(6), 444–455.

Faraone, S. V., & Antshel, K. M. (2014). Towards an evidence-based taxonomy of nonpharmacologic treatments for ADHD. *Child and Adolescent Psychiatric Clinics of North America, 23*(4), 965–972.

Gibbons, R. D., Weiss, D. J., Frank, E., & Kupfer, D. (2016). Computerized adaptive diagnosis and testing of mental health disorders. *Annual Review of Clinical Psychology, 12*, 83–104.

Holtmann, M., Sonuga-Barke, E., Cortese, S., & Brandeis, D. (2014). Neurofeedback for ADHD: A review of current evidence. *Child and Adolescent Psychiatric Clinics of North America, 23*(4), 789–806.

Livingstone, S., & Smith, P. K. (2014). Annual research review: Harms experienced by child users of online and mobile technologies: The nature, prevalence and management of sexual and aggressive risks in the digital age. *Journal of Child Psychology and Psychiatry and Allied Disciplines, 55*(6), 635–654.

Martin, D. M., McClintock, S. M., Forster, J., & Loo, C. K. (2016). Does therapeutic repetitive transcranial magnetic stimulation cause cognitive enhancing effects in patients with neuropsychiatric conditions?: A systematic review and meta-analysis of randomised controlled trials. *Neuropsychology Review, 26*(3), 295–309.

Motter, J. N., Pimontel, M. A., Rindskopf, D., Devanand, D. P., Doraiswamy, P. M., & Sneed, J. R. (2016). Computerized cognitive training and functional recovery in major depressive disorder: A meta-analysis. *Journal of Affective Disorders, 189*, 184–191.

Nikkelen, S. W., Valkenburg, P. M., Huizinga, M., & Bushman, B. J. (2014). Media use and ADHD-related behaviors in children and adolescents: A meta-analysis. *Developmental Psychology, 50*(9), 2228–2241.

Palm, U., Segmiller, F. M., Epple, A. N., Freisleder, F. J., Koutsouleris, N., Schulte-Körne, G., et al. (2016). Transcranial direct current stimulation in children and adolescents: A comprehensive review. *Journal of Neural Transmission, 123*, 1219–1234.

Perera, T., George, M. S., Grammer, G., Janicak, P. G., Pascual-Leone, A., & Wirecki, T. S. (2016). The clinical TMS Society consensus review and treatment recommendations for TMS therapy for major depressive disorder. *Brain Stimulation, 9*(3), 336–346.

Rubio, B., Boes, A. D., Laganiere, S., Rotenberg, A., Jeurissen, D., & Pascual-Leone, A. (2016). Noninvasive brain stimulation in pediatric attention-deficit hyperactivity disorder (ADHD): A review. *Journal of Child Neurology, 31*(6), 784–796.

CHAPTER 6: ENVIRONMENTAL CHEMICALS AND ADHD: SORTING ALARM FROM PRUDENT CAUTION

Arbuckle, T. E., Davis, K., Boylan, K., Fisher M., & Fu J. (2016). Bisphenol A, phthalates and lead and learning and behavioral problems in Canadian children 6–11 years of age: CHMS 2007–2009. *Neurotoxicology, 54*, 89–98.

Bell, M. R., Thompson, L. M., Rodriguez, K., & Gore, A. C. (2016). Two-hit exposure to polychlorinated biphenyls at gestational and juvenile life stages: 1. Sexually dimorphic effects on social and anxiety-like behaviors. *Hormones and Behavior, 78*, 168–177.

Bellinger, D. C. (2008). Very low lead exposures and children's neurodevelopment. *Current Opinion in Pediatrics, 20*(2), 172–177.

Bellinger, D. C. (2011). The protean toxicities of lead: New chapters in a familiar story. *International Journal of Environmental Research and Public Health, 8*(7), 2593–2628.

Berghuis, S. A., Bos, A. F., Sauer, P. J., & Roze, E. (2015). Developmental neurotoxicity of persistent organic pollutants: An update on childhood outcome. *Archives of Toxicology, 89,* 687–709.

Casas, M., Forns, J., Martínez, D., Avella-García, C., Valvi, D., Ballesteros-Gómez, A., et al. (2015). Exposure to bisphenol A during pregnancy and child neuropsychological development in the INMA-Sabadell cohort. *Environmental Research, 142,* 671–679.

Casati L., Sendra, R., Sibilia, V., & Celotti, F. (2015). Endocrine disrupters: The new players able to affect the epigenome. *Frontiers in Cell and Developmental Biology, 3,* 37.

Chopra, V., Harley, K., Lahiff, M., & Eskenazi, B. (2014). Association between phthalates and attention deficit disorder and learning disability in U.S. children 6–16 years. *Environmental Research, 128,* 64–69.

de Cock, M., Maas, Y. G., & van de Bor, M. (2012). Does perinatal exposure to endocrine disruptors induce autism spectrum and attention deficit hyperactivity disorders?: Review. *Acta Paediatrica, 101,* 811–818.

Engel, S. M., Wetmur, J., Chen, J., Zhu, C., Barr, D. B., Canfield, R. L., et al. (2011). Prenatal exposure to organophosphates, paraoxonase 1, and cognitive development in childhood. *Environmental Health Perspectives, 119*(8), 1182–1188.

Eriksson, U., & Kärrman, A. (2015). World-wide indoor exposure to polyfluoroalkyl phosphate esters (PAPs) and other PFASs in household dust. *Environmental Science and Technology, 49*(24), 14503–14511.

Eubig, P. A., Aguiar, A., & Schantz, S. L. (2010). Lead and PCBs as risk factors for attention deficit/hyperactivity disorder. *Environmental Health Perspectives, 118*(12), 1654–1667.

Evans, S. F., Kobrosly, R. W., Barrett, E. S., Thurston, S. W., Calafat, A. M., Weiss, B., et al. (2014). Prenatal bisphenol A exposure and maternally reported behavior in boys and girls. *Neurotoxicology, 45,* 91–99.

Gore, A. C., Chappell, V. A., Fenton, S. E., Flaws, J. A., Nadal, A., & Prins, G. S. (2015). Executive summary to EDC-2: The Endocrine Society's second scientific statement on endocrine-disrupting chemicals. *Endocrine Reviews, 36*(6), 593–602.

Gore, A. C., Chappell, V. A., Fenton, S. E., Flaws, J. A., Nadal, A., Prins, G. S., et al. (2015). EDC-2: The Endocrine Society's second scientific statement on endocrine-disrupting chemicals. *Endocrine Reviews, 36*(6), E1–E150.

Harley, K. G., Gunier, R. B., Kogut, K., Johnson, C., Bradman, A., Calafat, A. M., et al. (2013). Prenatal and early childhood bisphenol A concentrations and behavior in school-aged children. *Environmental Research, 126,* 43–50.

Holahan, M. R., & Smith, C. A. (2015). Phthalates and neurotoxic effects on hippocampal network plasticity. *Neurotoxicology, 48,* 21–34.

Hubbs-Tait, L., Nation, J. R., Krebs, N. F., & Bellinger, D. C. (2005). Neurotoxicants, micronutrients, and social environments: Individual and combined effects on children's development. *Psychological Science in the Public Interest*, 6(3), 57–121.

Landrigan, P. J. (2015). Children's environmental health: A brief history. *Academic Pediatrics*, 16(1), 1–9.

Lanphear, B. P. (2015). The impact of toxins on the developing brain. *Annual Review of Public Health*, 36, 211–230.

Livingstone, S., & Smith, P. K. (2014). Annual research review: Harms experienced by child users of online and mobile technologies: The nature, prevalence and management of sexual and aggressive risks in the digital age. *Journal of Child Psychology and Psychiatry and Allied Disciplines*, 55(6), 635–654.

Luo, M., Xu, Y., Cai, R., Tang, Y., Ge, M. M., Liu, Z. H., et al. (2014). Epigenetic histone modification regulates developmental lead exposure induced hyperactivity in rats. *Toxicology Letters*, 225(1), 78–85.

Mallozzi, M., Bordi, G., Garo, C., & Caserta, D. (2016). The effect of maternal exposure to endocrine disrupting chemicals on fetal and neonatal development: A review on the major concerns. *Birth Defects Research Part C: Embryo Today*, 108, 224–242.

Mustieles, V., Pérez-Lobato, R., Olea, N., & Fernández, M. F. (2015). Bisphenol A: Human exposure and neurobehavior. *Neurotoxicology*, 49, 174–184.

Nigg, J. T., Elmore, A. L., Natarajan, N., Friderici, K. H., & Nikolas, M. A. (2016). Variation in iron metabolism gene moderates the association between low-level blood lead exposure and attention-deficit/hyperactivity disorder. *Psychological Science*, 27, 257–269.

Nigg, J. T., Knottnerus, G. M., Martel, M. M., Nikolas, M., Cavanagh, K., Karmaus, W., et al. (2008). Low blood lead levels associated with clinically diagnosed attention deficit hyperactivity disorder (ADHD) and mediated by weak cognitive control. *Biological Psychiatry*, 63(3), 325–331.

Park, S., Lee, J. M., Kim, J. W., Cheong, J. H., Yun, H. J., Hong, Y. C., et al. (2015). Association between phthalates and externalizing behaviors and cortical thickness in children with attention deficit hyperactivity disorder. *Psychological Medicine*, 45(8), 1601–1612.

Pinson A., Bourguignon, J. P., & Parent, A. S. (2016). Exposure to endocrine disrupting chemicals and neurodevelopmental alterations. *Andrology*, 4(4), 706–722.

Richardson, J. R., Taylor, M. M., Shalat, S. L., Guillot, T. S., Caudle, W. M., Hossain, M. M., et al. (2015). Developmental pesticide exposure reproduces features of attention deficit hyperactivity disorder. *FASEB Journal*, 29(5), 1960–1972.

Stein, L. J., Gunier, R. B., Harley, K., Kogut, K., Bradman, A., & Eskenazi, B. (2016). Early childhood adversity potentiates the adverse association between prenatal organophosphate pesticide exposure and child IQ: The CHAMACOS cohort. *Neurotoxicology*, 56, 180–187.

Walker, D. M., & Gore, A. C. (2017). Epigenetic impacts of endocrine disruptors in the brain. *Frontiers of Neuroendocrinology*, 44, 1–26.

CHAPTER 7: ADVERSITY, STRESS, TRAUMA, AND ADHD: FINDING SANCTUARY

Beauchaine, T. P., Neuhaus, E., Zalewski, M., Crowell, S. E., & Potapova, N. (2011). The effects of allostatic load on neural systems subserving motivation, mood regulation, and social affiliation. *Developmental Psychopathology, 23*(4), 975–999.

Bethell, C. D., Newacheck, P., Hawes, E., & Halfon, N. (2014). Adverse childhood experiences: Assessing the impact on health and school engagement and the mitigating role of resilience. *Health Affairs, 33*(12), 2106–2115.

Biederman J., Petty, C., Spencer, T. J., Woodworth, K. Y., Bhide, P., Zhu J., et al. (2014). Is ADHD a risk for posttraumatic stress disorder (PTSD)?: Results from a large longitudinal study of referred children with and without ADHD. *World Journal of Biological Psychiatry, 15*(1), 49–55.

Cairncross M., & Miller, C.J. (2016). The effectiveness of mindfulness-based therapies for ADHD: A meta-analytic review. *Journal of Attention Disorders.* [Epub ahead of print]

Carey, B. (2016, May 29). Those with multiple tours of duty overseas struggle at home. *New York Times.* Retrieved from *www.nytimes.com/2016/05/30/health/veterans-iraq-afghanistan-psychology-therapy.html?_r=0.*

Carter, E. C., Pedersen, E. J., & McCullough, M. E. (2015). Reassessing intertemporal choice: Human decision-making is more optimal in a foraging task than in a self-control task. *Frontiers in Psychology, 6*(6), 95.

Coker, T. R., Elliott, M. N., Toomey, S. L., Schwebel, D. C., Cuccaro, P., Tortolero, S. R., et al. (2016). Racial and ethnic disparities in ADHD diagnosis and treatment. *Pediatrics, 138*(3), e20160407.

Felitti, V. J., Anda, R. F., Nordenberg, D., Williamson, D. F., Spitz, A. M., Edwards, V., et al. (1998). Relationship of childhood abuse and household dysfunction to many of the leading causes of death in adults: The Adverse Childhood Experiences (ACE) Study. *American Journal of Preventive Medicine, 14*(4), 245–258.

Finkelhor, D., Shattuck, A., Turner, H., & Hamby, S. (2013). Improving the adverse childhood experiences study scale. *Archives of Pediatric and Adolescent Medicine, 167*(1), 70–75.

Harrison, E. L., & Baune, B. T. (2014). Modulation of early stress-induced neurobiological changes: A review of behavioural and pharmacological interventions in animal models. *Translational Psychiatry, 4*(5), e390.

Horn, S. R., Charney, D. S., & Feder, A. (2016). Understanding resilience: New approaches for preventing and treating PTSD. *Experimental Neurology, 284*(Pt. B), 119–132.

Ieraci, A., Mallei, A., Musazzi, L., & Popoli, M. (2015). Physical exercise and acute restraint stress differentially modulate hippocampal brain-derived neurotrophic factor transcripts and epigenetic mechanisms in mice. *Hippocampus, 25*(11), 1380–1392.

Kallapiran, K., Koo, S., Kirubakaran, R., & Hancock, K. (2015). Effectiveness of mindfulness in improving mental health symptoms of children and adolescents: A meta-analysis. *Child and Adolescent Mental Health, 20,* 182–194.

Kashimoto, R. K., Toffoli, L. V., Manfredo, M. H., Volpini, V. L., Martins-Pinge, M. C., Pelosi, G. G., et al. (2016). Physical exercise affects the epigenetic programming of rat brain and modulates the adaptive response evoked by repeated restraint stress. *Behavioural Brain Research, 296,* 286–289.

Kennedy, M., Kreppner, J., Knights, N., Kumsta, R., Maughan, B., Golm, D., et al. (2016). Early severe institutional deprivation is associated with a persistent variant of adult attention-deficit/hyperactivity disorder. *Journal of Child Psychology and Psychiatry.* [Epub ahead of print]

Kuyken, W., Warren, F. C., Taylor, R. S., Whalley, B., Crane, C., Bondolfi, G., et al. (2016). Efficacy of mindfulness-based cognitive therapy in prevention of depressive relapse: An individual patient data meta-analysis from randomized trials. *JAMA Psychiatry,73*(6), 565–574.

McCauley, H. L., Breslau, J. A., Saito, N., & Miller, E. (2015). Psychiatric disorders prior to dating initiation and physical dating violence before age 21: Findings from the National Comorbidity Survey Replication (NCS-R). *Social Psychiatry and Psychiatric Epidemiology, 50*(9), 1357–1365.

Miller, T. W., Miller, R. A., & Nigg, J. T. (2009). Attention deficit/hyperactivity disorder in African American children: What can be concluded from the past ten years? *Clinical Psychology Review, 29,* 77–86.

Misiak, B., Frydecka, D., Zawadzki, M., Krefft, M., & Kiejna, A. (2014). Refining and integrating schizophrenia pathophysiology—relevance of the allostatic load concept. *Neuroscience and Biobehavioral Reviews, 45,* 183–201.

Moloney, R. D., Stilling, R. M., Dinan, T. G., & Cryan, J. F. (2015). Early-life stress-induced visceral hypersensitivity and anxiety behavior is reversed by histone deacetylase inhibition. *Neurogastroenterogy and Motility, 27*(12), 1831–1836.

Monk, C., Georgieff, M. K., & Osterholm, E. A. (2013). Research review: Maternal prenatal distress and poor nutrition—mutually influencing risk factors affecting infant neurocognitive development. *Journal of Child Psychology and Psychiatry and Allied Disciplines, 54*(2), 115–130.

Park, C. L. (2010). Making sense of the meaning literature: An integrative review of meaning making and its effects on adjustment to stressful life events. *Psychological Bulletin, 136,* 257–301.

Pastorelli, C., Lansford, J. E., Luengo, B. P., Malone, P. S., Di Giunta, L., Bacchini, D., et al. (2016). Positive parenting and children's prosocial behavior in eight countries. *Journal of Child Psychology and Psychiatry, 57,* 824–834.

Réus, G. Z., Abelaira, H. M., dos Santos, M. A., Carlessi, A. S., Tomaz, D. B., & Neotti, M. V. (2013). Ketamine and imipramine in the nucleus accumbens regulate histone deacetylation induced by maternal deprivation and are critical for associated behaviors. *Behavioural Brain Research, 256,* 451–456.

Rodrigues, G. M., Jr., Toffoli, L. V., Manfredo, M. H., Francis-Oliveira, J., Silva, A. S., Raquel, H. A., et al. (2015). Acute stress affects the global DNA methylation profile in rat brain: Modulation by physical exercise. *Behavioural Brain Research, 279,* 123–128.

Rutter, M. (2013). Annual research review: Resilience—clinical implications. *Journal of Child Psychology and Psychiatry, 54,* 474–487.

Spencer, A. E., Faraone, S. V., Bogucki, O. E., Pope, A. L., Uchida, M., Milad, M. R., et al. (2016). Examining the association between posttraumatic stress disorder and attention-deficit/hyperactivity disorder: A systematic review and meta-analysis. *Journal of Clinical Psychiatry, 77,* 72–83.

Spencer, S. J., Logel, C., & Davies, P. G. (2016). Stereotype threat. *Annual Review of Psychology, 67,* 415–438.

Stevens, J. R., & Stephens, D. W. (2010). The adaptive nature of impulsivity. In G. J. Madden & W. K. Bickel (Eds.), *Impulsivity: The behavioral and neurological science of discounting* (pp. 361–388). Washington, DC: American Psychological Association.

Stevens, S. E., Kumsta, R., Kreppner, J. M., Brookes, K. J., Rutter, M., & Sonuga-Barke, E. J. (2009). Dopamine transporter gene polymorphism moderates the effects of severe deprivation on ADHD symptoms: Developmental continuities in gene–environment interplay. *American Journal of Medical Genetics Part B: Neuropsychiatric Genetics, 150B(6),* 753–761.

Sturge-Apple, M., Suor, J. H., Davies, P. T., Cicchetti, D., Skibo, M. A., & Rogosch, F. A. (2016). Vagal tone and children's delay of gratification: Differential sensitivity in resource-poor and resource-rich environments. *Psychological Science, 27,* 885–894.

Teicher, M. H., & Samson, J. A. (2016). Annual research review: Enduring neurobiological effects of child abuse and neglect. *Journal of Child Psychology and Psychiatry, 57(3),* 241–266.

Werner, E. E. (2012). Children and war: Risk, resilience, and recovery. *Developmental Psychopathology, 24,* 553–558.

Wu, G., Feder, A., Cohen, H., Kim, J. J., Calderon, S., Charney, D. S., et al. (2013). Understanding resilience. *Frontiers in Behavioral Neuroscience, 7,* 1–15.

CHAPTER 8: GETTING PROFESSIONAL HELP: TRADITIONAL AND ALTERNATIVE TREATMENTS FOR ADHD

Arns, M., Loo, S. K., Sterman, M. B., Heinrich, H., Kuntsi, J., Asherson, P., et al. (2016). Editorial perspective: How should child psychologists and psychiatrists interpret FDA device approval? Caveat emptor. *Journal of Child Psychology and Psychiatry, 57(5),* 656–658.

Berman, S. M., Kuczenski, R., McCracken, J. T., & London, E. D. (2009). Potential adverse effects of amphetamine treatment on brain and behavior: A review. *Molecular Psychiatry, 14(2),* 123–142.

Bledsoe, J., Semrud-Clikeman, M., & Pliszka, S. R. (2009). A magnetic resonance imaging study of the cerebellar vermis in chronically treated and treatment-naïve children with attention-deficit/ hyperactivity disorder combined type. *Biological Psychiatry, 65(7),* 620–624.

Bloch, M. H. (2012). Misplaced fear?: FDA contraindication to psychostimulant use in children with tics. *Evidence-Based Child Health, 7(4),* 1231–1234.

Cameron, S., Glyde, H., Dillon, H., King, A., & Gillies, K. (2015). Results from a National Central Auditory Processing Disorder Service: A real-world assessment of diagnostic practices and remediation for central auditory processing disorder. *Seminars in Hearing, 36*(4), 216–236.

Castellanos, F. X., & Meyer, E. (2013). Toward systems neuroscience of shared and distinct neural effects of medications used to treat attention-deficit/hyperactivity disorder. *Biological Psychiatry, 74*(8), 560–562.

Cheng, C. H., Chan, P. Y., Hsieh, Y. W., & Chen, K. F. (2016). A meta-analysis of mismatch negativity in children with attention deficit-hyperactivity disorders. *Neuroscience Letters, 612*, 132–137.

Coghill, D., Banaschewski, T., Zuddas, A., Pelaz A., Gagliano A., & Doepfner, M. (2013). Long-acting methylphenidate formulations in the treatment of attention-deficit/hyperactivity disorder: A systematic review of head-to-head studies. *BMC Psychiatry, 13*, 237.

Comim, C. M., Gomes, K. M., Réus, G. Z., Petronilho, F., Ferreira, G. K., Streck, E. L., et al. (2014). Methylphenidate treatment causes oxidative stress and alters energetic metabolism in an animal model of attention-deficit hyperactivity disorder. *Acta Neuropsychiatrica, 26*(2), 96–103.

Daley, D., van der Oord, S., Ferrin, M., Danckaerts, M., Doepfner, M., Cortese, S., et al. (2014). Behavioral interventions in attention-deficit/hyperactivity disorder: A meta-analysis of randomized controlled trials across multiple outcome domains. *Journal of the American Academy of Child and Adolescent Psychiatry, 53*(8), 835–847.

DeBonis, D. A. (2015). It is time to rethink central auditory processing disorder protocols for school-aged children. *American Journal of Audiology, 24*(2), 124–136.

DuPaul, G. J., Gormley, M. J., & Laracy, S. D. (2014). School-based interventions for elementary school students with ADHD. *Child and Adolescent Psychiatric Clinics of North America, 23*(4), 687–697.

Evans, S. W., Langberg, J. M., Egan, T., & Molitor, S. J. (2014). Middle school-based and high school-based interventions for adolescents with ADHD. *Child and Adolescent Psychiatric Clinics of North America, 23*(4), 699–715.

Fagundes, A. O., Aguiar, M. R., Aguiar, C. S., Scaini, G., Sachet, M. U., & Bernhardt, N. M. (2010). Effect of acute and chronic administration of methylphenidate on mitochondrial respiratory chain in the brain of young rats. *Neurochemical Research, 35*(11), 1675–1680.

Fumagalli, F., Cattaneo, A., Caffino, L., Ibba, M., Racagni, G., Carboni, E., et al. (2010). Sub-chronic exposure to atomoxetine up-regulates BDNF expression and signalling in the brain of adolescent spontaneously hypertensive rats: Comparison with methylphenidate. *Pharmacological Research, 62*(6), 523–529.

Gill, K. E., Pierre, P. J., Daunais, J., Bennett, A. J., Martelle, S., Gage, H. D., et al. (2012). Chronic treatment with extended release methylphenidate does not alter dopamine systems or increase vulnerability for cocaine self-administration: A study in nonhuman primates. *Neuropsychopharmacology, 37*(12), 2555–2565.

Haack, L. M., Villodas, M., McBurnett, K., Hinshaw, S., & Pfiffner, L. J. (2016). Parenting as a mechanism of change in psychosocial treatment for youth with ADHD, predominantly inattentive presentation. *Journal of Abnormal Child Psychology*. [Epub ahead of print]

Harstad, E. B., Weaver, A. L., Katusic, S. K., Colligan, R. C., Kumar, S., Chan, E., et al. (2014). ADHD, stimulant treatment, and growth: A longitudinal study. *Pediatrics, 134*(4), e935–e944.

Heine C., & O'Halloran, R. J. (2015). Central auditory processing disorder: A systematic search and evaluation of clinical practice guidelines. *Journal of Evaluation in Clinical Practice, 21*(6), 988–994.

Hinshaw, S. P., Arnold, L. E., & MTA Cooperative Group. (2015). Attention-deficit hyperactivity disorder, multimodal treatment, and longitudinal outcome: Evidence, paradox, and challenge. *Wiley Interdisciplinary Reviews: Cognitive Science, 6*(1), 39–52.

Millichap, J. G. (2015). Risk of tics with psychostimulants for ADHD. *Pediatric Neurology Briefs, 29*(12), 95.

Ollendick, T. H., Greene, R. W., Fraire, M. G., Austin, K. E., Halldorsdottir, T., Allen, K. B., et al. (2016). Parent Management Training (PMT) and Collaborative & Proactive Solutions (CPS) in the treatment of oppositional defiant disorder in youth: A randomized control trial. *Journal of Clinical Child and Adolescent Psychology, 45,* 591–604.

Pfiffner, L. J., & Haack, L. M. (2014). Behavior management for school-aged children with ADHD. *Child and Adolescent Psychiatric Clinics of North America, 23*(4), 731–746.

Poulton, A. S., Bui, Q., Melzer, E., & Evans, R. (2016). Stimulant medication effects on growth and bone age in children with attention-deficit/hyperactivity disorder: A prospective cohort study. *International Clinical Psychopharmacology, 31*(2), 93–99.

Pringsheim, T., & Steeves, T. (2011). Pharmacological treatment for Attention Deficit Hyperactivity Disorder (ADHD) in children with comorbid tic disorders. *Cochrane Database of Systematic Reviews, 4,* CD007990.

Sadasivan, S., Pond, B. B., Pani, A. K., Qu, C., Jiao, Y., & Smeyne, R. J. (2012). Methylphenidate exposure induces dopamine neuron loss and activation of microglia in the basal ganglia of mice. *PLoS ONE, 7*(3), e33693.

Schmitz, F., Scherer, E. B., Machado, F. R., da Cunha, A. A., Tagliari, B., Netto, C. A., et al. (2012). Methylphenidate induces lipid and protein damage in prefrontal cortex, but not in cerebellum, striatum and hippocampus of juvenile rats. *Metabolic Brain Disease, 27*(4), 605–612.

Schnoebelen, S., Semrud-Clikeman, M., & Pliszka, S. R. (2010). Corpus callosum anatomy in chronically treated and stimulant naïve ADHD. *Journal of Attention Disorders, 14*(3), 256–266.

Simchon, Y., Weizman, A., & Rehavi, M. (2010). The effect of chronic methylphenidate administration on presynaptic dopaminergic parameters in a rat model for ADHD. *European Neuropsychopharmacology, 20*(10), 714–720.

Simchon-Tenenbaum, Y., Weizman, A., & Rehavi, M. (2015a). Alterations in brain neurotrophic and glial factors following early age chronic methylphenidate and cocaine administration. *Behavioural Brain Research, 282,* 125–132.

Simchon-Tenenbaum, Y., Weizman, A., & Rehavi, M. (2015b). The impact of chronic early administration of psychostimulants on brain expression of

BDNF and other neuroplasticity-relevant proteins. *Journal of Molecular Neuroscience, 57*(2), 231–242.

Snyder, S. M., Rugino, T. A., Hornig, M., & Stein, M. A. (2015). Integration of an EEG biomarker with a clinician's ADHD evaluation. *Brain and Behavior, 5*(4), e00330.

Spencer, T. J., Brown, A., Seidman, L. J., Valera, E. M., Makris, N., Lomedico, A., et al. (2013) Effect of psychostimulants on brain structure and function in ADHD: A qualitative literature review of magnetic resonance imaging-based neuroimaging studies. *Journal of Clinical Psychiatry, 74*, 902–917.

Stein, M. A., Snyder, S. M., Rugino, T. A., & Hornig, M. (2016). Commentary: Objective aids for the assessment of ADHD—further clarification of what FDA approval for marketing means and why NEBA might help clinicians: A response to Arns et al. (2016). *Journal of Child Psychology and Psychiatry, 57*(6), 770–771.

Urban, K. R., Waterhouse, B. D., & Gao, W. J. (2012). Distinct age-dependent effects of methylphenidate on developing and adult prefrontal neurons. *Biological Psychiatry, 72*(10), 880–888.

van der Marel, K., Bouet, V., Meerhoff, G. F., Freret, T., Boulouard, M., Dauphin, F., et al. (2015). Effects of long-term methylphenidate treatment in adolescent and adult rats on hippocampal shape, functional connectivity and adult neurogenesis. *Neuroscience, 309*, 243–258.

Villemonteix, T., De Brito, S. A., Kavec, M., Balériaux, D., Metens, T., Slama, H., et al. (2015). Grey matter volumes in treatment naïve vs. chronically treated children with attention deficit/hyperactivity disorder: A combined approach. *European Neuropsychopharmacology, 25*(8), 1118–1127.

Wang, G. J., Volkow, N. D., Wigal, T., Kollins, S. H., Newcorn, J. H., Telang, F., et al. (2013). Long-term stimulant treatment affects brain dopamine transporter level in patients with attention deficit/hyperactive disorder. *PLoS ONE, 8*(5), e63023.

Index

About the Author

Joel T. Nigg, PhD, is Professor of Psychiatry and Behavioral Neuroscience at Oregon Health & Science University. A leading expert on ADHD, he has conducted scientific research and worked with children and their families on diagnostic assessment and treatment planning since the 1990s. His website is *www.guilford.com/joel-nigg*.